A Town Called Asbestos

The Nature | History | Society series is devoted to the publication of high-quality scholarship in environmental history and allied fields. Its broad compass is signalled by its title: nature because it takes the natural world seriously; history because it aims to foster work that has temporal depth; and society because its essential concern is with the interface between nature and society, broadly conceived. The series is avowedly interdisciplinary and is open to the work of anthropologists, ecologists, historians, geographers, literary scholars, political scientists, sociologists, and others whose interests resonate with its mandate. It offers a timely outlet for lively, innovative, and well-written work on the interaction of people and nature through time in North America.

General Editor: Graeme Wynn, University of British Columbia

A list of titles in the series appears at the end of the book.

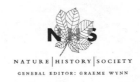

NATURE | HISTORY | SOCIETY
GENERAL EDITOR: GRAEME WYNN

A Town
Called Asbestos

Environmental Contamination, Health, and Resilience in a Resource Community

JESSICA VAN HORSSEN

FOREWORD BY GRAEME WYNN

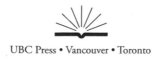

UBC Press • Vancouver • Toronto

25 24 23 22 21 20 19 18 17 16   5 4 3 2 1

Printed in Canada on FSC-certified ancient-forest-free paper
(100% post-consumer recycled) that is processed chlorine- and acid-free.

Library and Archives Canada Cataloguing in Publication

van Horssen, Jessica, author
    A town called Asbestos : environmental contamination, health, and resilience in a resource community / Jessica van Horssen.

(Nature, history, society)
Includes bibliographical references and index.
Issued in print and electronic formats.
ISBN 978-0-7748-2841-3 (bound). – ISBN 978-0-7748-2843-7 (pdf)
ISBN 978-0-7748-2844-4 (epub)

    1. Asbestos (Québec). 2. Asbestos (Québec) – History. 3. Asbestos (Québec) – Economic conditions. 4. Asbestos mines and mining – Québec (Province) – Asbestos. 5. Asbestos mines and mining – Environmental aspects – Québec (Province) – Asbestos. 6. Asbestos mines and mining – Health aspects – Québec (Province) – Asbestos. Asbestos industry – Québec (Province) – Asbestos. 8. Asbestos industry – Political aspects – Québec (Province) – Asbestos. I. Title. II. Series: Nature, history, society

FC2949.A82V35 2016   971.4'573   C2015-905843-0
                                                               C2015-905844-9

Canadä

UBC Press gratefully acknowledges the financial support for our publishing program of the Government of Canada (through the Canada Book Fund), the Canada Council for the Arts, and the British Columbia Arts Council.

This book has been published with the help of a grant from the Canadian Federation for the Humanities and Social Sciences, through the Awards to Scholarly Publications Program, using funds provided by the Social Sciences and Humanities Research Council of Canada.

UBC Press
The University of British Columbia
2029 West Mall
Vancouver, BC V6T 1Z2
www.ubcpress.ca

Contents

Illustrations

The Long Dying

Graeme Wynn

THE TENTH VOLUME in a highly acclaimed series of crime-fiction stories by Quebec author Louise Penny begins with former police inspector Armand Gamache settling into his retirement. Living happily in a modest village nestled in the forested, rolling hills between Quebec and Vermont, he revels in morning walks with his wife and dog, and the pleasure of sitting on a hilltop bench to read in the sunshine. Occasionally, he takes the opportunity to gaze down at the settlement of Three Pines below, huddled next the river, "as though held in the palm of an ancient hand. A stigmata in the Québec countryside. Not a wound, but a wonder." Readers of *The Long Way Home* soon learn that the Gamache house fronts on to the little green of this picturesque village. Clad in white clapboard with a large verandah in front, and a terrace and large neglected garden out back, it is something of a magnet in the social life of Three Pines. Here Armand and Reine-Marie entertain friends, inviting them on summer Friday afternoons to settle into Adirondack chairs on the lawn and enjoy white wine and morsels of "smoked trout on rye." Then, as dusk arrives, tea lamps are lit, making it appear as though "large fireflies had settled in for the evening." The village had "the rhythm, the cadence, of a piece of music." So much was right with this world that even weeds became glories: the "tall, effusive bouquet" that brightened the inside of the Gamaches' home was made of purple loosestrife, bishop's weed, and bindweed.[1]

This idyll was not for long, however. Asked by a neighbour for help in locating her estranged artist husband, Gamache embarks on a journey that carries him into the province's harsh backcountry and brings him face to face with the heart of darkness. On a boat along the St. Lawrence, bound for the lower North Shore ("A coast so forbidding, so hostile it was fit only for the damned"), the detective and his companions begin to suspect a devious plot to cause death by unconventional means, when a white powder is discovered in a tube that once held a painting or a blank canvas.[2] The air of fundamental decency and goodness associated with Three Pines gives way to a sense of iniquity and terror as the detective identifies the substance and quizzes a young science teacher on her way to Blanc Sablon about its properties.

Suspecting that the powder might be asbestos, the group learns that it is dangerous if inhaled. "How long does it take to kill someone?" they ask. "Depends," says the teacher, "it does take a while for the effects to be noticed." Well then, said Gamache, "would the person necessarily die, if he inhaled it?" Immediately concerned, the teacher looked quizzically at her interrogators. "No," Gamache smiled reassuringly. "But if we had, then what? Would we die?" Hmmm, said the teacher, "you might. It's one of those tricks of fate. Not all asbestos miners developed lung disease. Some people exposed only incidentally did." And so the questions continued, until Gamache summed up what he had learned: "Asbestos is deadly. " Nothing was certain, "but there was a pretty good chance that whoever handled ... [the] asbestos-infected paintings would inhale it and eventually die." Earlier, an Internet search for information about the substance had revealed that "it had seemed a godsend to a hardscrabble region [of Quebec where it was mined]. Natural, plentiful. It was both an insulator and a fire retardant. Asbestos would save the region and save lives. It was magic." But it was not enchantment that Gamache confronted on his journey into another hardscrabble region, the territory described by John Cabot as the land God gave to Cain; it was murder, the very crime for which Cain had been cursed by God.[3]

Asbestos intrudes into Louise Penny's book as a mysterious, toxic substance, but it is more important as an idea that helps knit together good and evil, magic and malevolence, despair and redemption, brokenness and grace. It augments and amplifies the message of the little volume that Gamache reads on his hilltop bench: "There is a balm in Gilead,/To make the wounded whole./There's power enough in Heaven, / To cure a sin-sick soul."[4] For Jessica van Horssen, by contrast, asbestos is both a material substance (fibrous chrysotile, the progenitor of the deadly powder that worried the detective so) and (with a capital A) a real place, a town called Asbestos, not far from Gamache's Three Pines in the *Estrie* (Eastern Townships) region of Quebec. Her book knits these two versions of asbestos together into an arresting and important account of how economic, political, geological, and social circumstances, the restraint of information, and the denial of risk led to the long slow death of a community and many of its people.

A Town Called Asbestos is, quite remarkably, the first book-length study to consider the environmental history and geography of this storied and troubled place. Rooted in government and corporate archival sources, local newspaper reports, and town council minutes, as well as a rich array of other reports and published material, the volume before you traverses the blurred boundaries between humans and the natural environment, and explores, to revealing effect, "the intimacy between life and labour" in a single-resource town. It details how residents of Asbestos thought of themselves and their community and fought – proudly and staunchly – for the survival of both through the rise and fall of the industry on which they depended. But it is also unflinching in revealing how many of those who struggled and persisted here against great odds fell prey, in time, to asbestos-related diseases, the full effects of which remained undisclosed for decades after they were known. Measuring their circumstances against the comfort Gamache found in the Gilead refrain, it is sobering to recognize that ignorance was the only balm available to these "unknowing test mice in a giant living laboratory," the sick and wounded souls of *A Town Called Asbestos,* few of whom would ever be made whole again (van Horssen, this volume).

By describing Three Pines as a wonder, Gamache encourages us to think of Asbestos, by contrast, as a stigmatic wound marking the bodies of the land, people, and society that provide the central axes of van Horssen's account of this part of eastern Quebec. Here, rolling Appalachian hills once clothed by forest are ripped asunder in the quest for chrysotile, and a mammoth open pit, thousands of metres in circumference and hundreds deep, is expanded inexorably to consume parts of the town housing those who work its depths. Here people carry the signs of close and prolonged exposure to asbestos fibre, signs often undetected and unrecognized until the coughing and shortness of breath that might have a dozen causes are identified by medical science as marks of mesothelioma or asbestosis. Here too, in this story of resource exploitation, society bears the consequences of inadequate regulation in a world devoted to economic expansion built on the bedrock of corporate profits. These are the marks of the Western world's crown of thorns.

This is a compelling story. It has never been told in quite this way or, specifically, for this particular place. But it is also, at base, an old and familiar tale, one that draws on and echoes prominent and recurring themes in the environmental (and economic and social) history of the modern world. Van Horssen's interest is clearly focused on Asbestos, but her account – which engages broad intellectual horizons and sharpens understanding of the human condition – ranges widely across disciplines, their literatures, and the face of the earth. This is the story of a town, its people, and its major industry. But the nature of that industry created environmental problems for the town; afflicted its citizens with illnesses that were the focus of a growing body of international medical research; linked this small place in Quebec to communities elsewhere through commodity chains and corporate ties; and embroiled Asbestos, its citizens, the Johns-Manville company, and eventually the governments of Quebec and Canada, in a global debate about the morality of continuing to utilize asbestos. This, then, is a timely reminder that the modern world is a tangled web of connections among farms, factories and consumers, companies and politicians, actions and reactions, and that – as environmental historian Brett Walker has noted in his book on the toxic archipelago of Japan – "our lives depend on these relationships – and are imperiled by them as well."[5]

A half century and more ago, Rachel Carson drew attention to the toxic implications of one of these interconnections – the slow build-up of synthetic chemical pesticides in the bodies of living beings. Developed by scientists to kill pests that ravaged crops and spread disease, these substances (such as DDT) did exactly the work for which they were intended but much more besides as they entered the food chain. Because most pesticides are relatively persistent in the environment (DDT has a half-life of fifteen years), Carson argued that their indiscriminate use would have lasting and detrimental effects as the twinned processes of bioaccumulation and biomagnification raised their concentrations to levels that were fatal to birds and fish and threatened human health.[6]

Silent Spring, the book that brought this message to the world, drew its title from a poem by John Keats and began with a wonderful evocative essay that both encapsulated and distorted its essential argument.[7] "There was once a town in the heart of America where all life seemed to live in harmony with its surroundings," wrote Carson in "A Fable for Tomorrow." Species-rich forests, "great ferns and wildflowers," birds and fish in abundance, foxes barking in the hills, and deer "half hidden in the mists of the fall mornings" as they ghosted across the checkerboard of fields that surrounded prosperous farms, these were the elements of this calm and pleasant place, just as they had been since the first settlers arrived many years before. But they were no more. A "strange blight [had] crept over the area," animals sickened and died, farmers and their families took ill, and a strange stillness lay over the land as no birds sang. Neither witchcraft nor enemy action had caused this transformation. "The people had done it themselves." Earlier in the year they had sprayed a "white granular powder" that fell "like snow upon the roofs and the lawns, the fields and streams." Mere weeks had turned that fair town in the heart of America from idyll to wasteland, from wonder to wound.

But the stillness that Carson feared and anticipated to such telling effect would not envelop the land overnight. DDT is sub-lethal to species other than insects, and its effects on bird populations are felt through shell-thinning and reproductive failure rather than sudden, mass death. *Silent Spring* is about the long-game; it deals with slow-moving processes that work incrementally to produce calamitous repercussions on a time scale stretching across years and decades. Carson's "Fable" is a powerful caution emphasizing the "grim specter" of environmental harm caused by human hubris – but it compresses time to achieve its effect. Faced with the challenge of portraying the "pervasive but elusive" consequences of what literary scholar Rob Nixon calls "slow violence" – by which he means the ravages wrought by climate change, deforestation, the aftermaths of oil spills, the release of radioactive substances into the atmosphere, and other slowly unfolding environmental crises – Carson used her fable as an opening gambit, to drive home the essence rather than the specific substance of her argument.[8]

Asbestos, the substance, perpetrated slow violence in Asbestos, the town – as well as in many other locations beyond – and van Horssen's book contributes, quietly, to understanding the workings of that insidious process that Nixon characterizes "from a narrative perspective" as "invisible, mutagenic theater ... slow-paced but open-ended" and lacking "the tidy closure ... imposed by the visual orthodoxies of victory and defeat."[9] *A Town Called Asbestos* is, in essence, an account of the exposure of relatively poor and politically marginalized people to the slow-acting ravages of almost invisible fibres that degrade many of their bodies and generate a sense of uncertainty and foreboding about the future. It is the story of local economies, communities, and ecologies subject to the slings and arrows of fluctuating fortunes dictated by distant markets, remote corporate leaders, and politicians from afar. Through these pages we come to understand one of the cruel ironies that Nixon associates with slow violence: that it mostly goes unremarked, first because it is incremental in effect and complicated to explain, which makes it a difficult subject for media that "venerate the spectacular" and prefer "sound-bite" explanations;

and second, because its very gradualness takes it off the radar of politicians and policy makers focused on the immediate and newsworthy. Centred though they are in eastern Quebec, the developments traced here also reveal that slow violence is generally as much the consequence of choice as of time – that few things "just happen," and that the courses on which events unfold always depend, to some degree, on the decisions and (in)actions of those involved in them.

Silent Spring was a landmark book, one of the most important pieces of environmental writing ever produced. It did much to change North American attitudes toward nature, driving home the fundamental ecological message that everything is connected to everything else, crystallizing emergent concerns about the systemic spread of radioactive substances, such as Strontium 90; the damaging effects of new drugs, such as thalidomide; and spawning the modern environmental movement.[10] For its admirers, it "altered the balance of power in the world," and ensured that "no one since would be able to sell pollution as the necessary underside of progress so easily or uncritically."[11] But there are limits to what any book can do, and the history recounted in *A Town Called Asbestos* suggests that admiration for Carson's achievements should be less sanguine.[12]

One of the most chastening observations to fall from Rob Nixon's reading of postcolonial literature from an environmental perspective, and the close linkage between environmental degradation and the oppression of the poor revealed by this, is that "slow violence provides prevaricative cover for the forces that have the most to profit from inaction."[13] Reflecting on the ways in which this occurred in the global south over the last thirty years, Nixon notes that deception and misrepresentation have been integral to the evasive tactics that have created space to stall. Here he has the doubt-disseminators of Big Oil, Big Coal, and Big Tobacco firmly in his sights – the lobbyists, consultants, media plutocrats, and right-wing think-tanks that deal in ambiguous, confusing, and false information to create a climate conducive to inaction. These are the "bewilderers," those whom Frantz Fanon saw standing alongside self-proclaimed moral teachers and counselors to "separate the exploited from those in power" in capitalist countries, much as the policeman and the soldier, the rifle butt and napalm, served to segregate natives from settlers in the colonies.[14] In Asbestos, the deceptions may have been less complete, less blatant, and less orchestrated than those choreographed by merchants of doubt in the neoliberal world order.[15] But Johns-Manville; their local white-collar employees; and municipal, provincial, and federal politicians all found some benefit, and a degree of cover, in the claim that some level of pollution was an inescapable consequence of maintaining jobs and profits (and the often less-than-forceful actions to minimize it that ensued).

Pathos and tragedy are significant themes in van Horssen's history of Asbestos but they are not all she wrote. There are important positive dimensions to this story, which endows the people of the community with that most fundamental and admirable of human characteristics: resilience. Against the odds, in the face of difficulties and indignities of various sorts, they battled on. At times they were misguided; at others, in stubborn denial of what others could see and believed to be against their best interests. But the mine meant work, a paycheque, and the chance to own a house and enjoy the comforts of home. As Gamache learned, these things "seemed a godsend" in this hardscrabble region. Even after much had gone sour, jobs were lost, and the long-term effects of asbestos exposure were clearly evident in elevated cancer rates and newly public medical reports, long-time residents were reluctant to deny the magic that asbestos had wrought in the area. In 1997, four men from the community ran a marathon in France to show that there was nothing wrong with their lungs, and a decade after that many townspeople rallied against changing the name of the town to Trois Lacs or Phoenix because they felt that to do so would be to "tell the world that we are ashamed of our product."

Naïve, poignant, even pitiable though they may seem, such gestures are important because they force us to ask "Why?" Reading *A Town Called Asbestos* and wondering why people delude themselves in the face of overwhelming evidence challenging their convictions, we might find some explanation in the importance society attaches to getting ahead or hanging on – to self-reliance. And we might extend this thread to reflect on the power of expectations, on the way "responsibilities" are ingrained and shaped by prevailing discourse and so on.

Asking "Why?" again, we might ponder the moral and emotional dimensions of this story without reducing it to the sort of high melodrama that turns on simplified versions of the actors and the issues. Indeed, there are complex, difficult matters at stake here. As other studies have noted, failures to recognize and act on the deleterious effects of the mineral are not always wilful. Asbestos fibres are microscopic – "one million fibrils can be lined up in one inch" – and their impact on human health remains latent for decades. But van Horssen makes it clear that the silences surrounding asbestos pollution in Quebec cannot be attributed largely or entirely to such "material constraints." There is ample evidence that institutional inertia, corporate concealment, and a weak regulatory environment allowed the asbestos hazard to go unaddressed far longer than might or ought to have been the case. So, for example, Johns-Manville company officials, unwilling to sacrifice profits for the health of workers, insisted that they could control the asbestos dust problem, and no health officials insisted on rigorous scrutiny of their claims.[16] But why, we must ask, were opportunities for such behaviour created and then allowed to prevail? Why is it that companies have been able to put profits before people (and the environment) in their calculus of significance? Might it have anything to do with the observation, made by van Horssen, that effective campaigns against asbestos only began when Western society came to understand the risks it posed to the public at large—and the implication that some people – miners? the poor? – are "disposable," or hardly worth society's concern?

Finally, this book might lead readers to ask why, in a country as affluent as Canada, politicians and governments were willing to dissemble and deny to keep asbestos production afloat. Why were national and provincial leaders willing to stand on the world stage and deflect pressures to stop extraction, or pretend that Canadian asbestos really was magically "inert" and benign, when this meant risking, if not literally sacrificing, the lives of citizens? Surely there were alternatives. Then as now, it was and is inappropriate to defer to the economy, profits, and prosperity as the reasons for inaction. We should not forget that the long dyings continue. A recent report in the *Globe and Mail* noted that "about 152,000" Canadian workers are currently exposed to asbestos and that such exposure was "the single largest on-the-job killer in Canada, accounting for more than a third of total workplace death claims approved last year [i.e., 2013] and nearly a third since 1996."[17] Other countries have banned asbestos just as they have acted more decisively than has Canada on a number of other vexing environmental and social-justice concerns. Should not this story of asbestos in Quebec lead us to ask whether there are parallels in the ongoing development of the oil and gas industry in Western Canada even as scientific evidence of the global perils of greenhouse gas emissions mounts, and there are troubling signs of detrimental health outcomes for residents downstream and downwind of the oil sands?

Recognizing that deception and misunderstanding are important elements of *The Long Way Home*, even as its plot turns on the ways in which artists (and others) can lose their souls in the pursuit of greatness, one reviewer found a lesson in that book. "Those who manage to find a balm for their past wounds, move forward in their lives." Pain and struggle may persist but they are able to "keep walking on into the light of a new and brighter day." By contrast, "those who cling to the scars of the past die in the shadows."[18] In the assessment of another reader, Gamache drew his own life lesson from his long career in the Sûreté du Québec: "People must be saved … from the brutality of others and sometimes from themselves."[19] Both, it seems to me, are lessons reaffirmed in the pages of *A Town Called Asbestos*, and they and this book are worth reading (and remembering) for that, as we grapple with what Edward Said once called "the normalized quiet of unseen power."[20]

Acknowledgments

THE RESEARCHING AND writing of this book would not have been possible without the unwavering support of new acquaintances, respected scholars, and old friends. Key contacts in Asbestos were John Millen at the Musée minéralogique d'Asbestos and G. Claude Théroux at the Société d'Histoire d'Asbestos. Both of these men provided invaluable sources and insight into the community, inspiring me to look deeper into the past and question my own assumptions about people and place. The staff at the Hôtel de ville d'Asbestos were also accommodating and helped broaden my understanding of how the community operated in the past and in the present.

Beyond Asbestos, the archivists and commissionaires at the Bibliothèque et Archives nationals du Québec made researching in Quebec City fully entertaining, and Jean-Pierre Kesteman directed me to key resources on the early history of Asbestos. Dr. David Egilman first introduced me to the wealth of historical information at Johns-Manville's Asbestos Claims Research Facility and helped bring new context and meaning to this study. Geoffrey Tweedale followed suit, and I appreciated the hospitality he and his wife Mary showed me in Manchester just as much as the sources he provided. Both Egilman and Tweedale took an interest in my study that encouraged me throughout the research and writing process. This book would not be what it is without their generosity. Maggie Baumgardner at the Johns-Manville Asbestos Claims Research Facility was also helpful in gaining permission to use many of the vital sources I employ.

Jean Manore at Bishop's University was the first to inspire me to pursue graduate studies, and Chad Gaffield and Michael Behiels at the University of Ottawa further inspired my dedication to the field. I also had a great amount of help from my doctoral supervisor, Alan MacEachern, who challenged me to look at my subject and my role as historian from new perspectives. His consideration and patience were greatly appreciated. In addition, I was fortunate to have a community of scholars around me at the University of Western Ontario and through the Network in Canadian History and Environment, including Shelley McKellar, Robert Wardhaugh, William J. Turkel, Stéphane Castonguay, Joanna Dean, and Graeme Wynn. During my postdoctoral fellowship at McGill University and the Université du Québec à Trois-Rivières, Stéphane Castonguay, Stéphan Gervais, Mary Anne Poutanen, Jarrett Rudy, and Suzanne Morton brought me into a wonderful community of scholars that continues to inspire me and enrich my work. My time teaching at York University added to my list of wonderful colleagues and scholars who have encouraged me throughout the process of writing this book, including Sean Kheraj, Jennifer Stephens, Molly Ladd-Taylor, Marcel Martel, Deb Neill, and Craig Heron. All of these scholars encouraged me to think and write about Asbestos from new angles. Of particular note is Joy Parr, who taught me to trust my instincts as an historian and motivated me to always think creatively, compassionately, and constructively. I would not be the scholar I am today without her guidance, encouragement, and strength.

Graeme Wynn was relentless in encouraging me to make this book the best it could be, and through his sharp editorial eye, made this work – and my writing – significantly better than it was. I have learned so much from him. Randy Schmidt at UBC Press was also a privilege to work with, as he put just enough pressure and humour into the process to motivate me. My friends and family have been heroically understanding for the duration of this project, acting as sounding boards, cheerleaders, proofreaders, and chefs. Radha-Prema Paquette brought this book to life through her illustrations of the graphic novel based on my research (http://megaprojects. uwo.ca/asbestos/) and helped me keep my sanity with sauciness and a genuine interest in rocks. I will never forget our time eating cherries in the sun. The generosity of Ang and Rich Waterton continues to astound me, and I will never be able to thank them enough for putting a roof over my head, food in my stomach, and laughter in my heart. The Lost Boys of Lavington Court could not have been more wonderful. Or hilarious. Shannon Hodge and Jason Hughes were my Montreal champions, always willing to take an interest in whatever thoughts on Asbestos were rambling in my head at the time. Rebecca Jane Woods and Teresa Iacobelli have been comrades in the academic trenches and very dear friends, as have Priya Raju and Sarah Doran, dear friends who possess a startling confidence in my abilities and continue to be an inexhaustible source of motivation. My parents, Frank and Theresa, have supported me throughout this project and taught me fundamental life lessons while showing unimagined patience and love for their stressed-out daughter. My Oma, Johanna, offered support, motivation, and ice cream throughout this process and remains my sunshine on a cloudy day. With his genuine fascination in all things under the sun, my partner Alexander Hall helped me think more deeply and more constructively about this study and my role as a scholar with his amazing ability to put everything in perspective, especially when the process of writing this book seemed insurmountable. All of these people now know far more about Asbestos than they probably ever hoped to, and without them, this work would not be complete and I would not be where I am today.

Abbreviations

ACRF	Asbestos Claims Research Facility
BAL Co.	British American Land Company
BANQ	Bibliothèque et Archives Nationales du Québec
CGS	Canadian Geological Survey
C-JM	Canadian Johns-Manville
CLC	Canadian Labour Congress
CMAJ	Canadian Medical Association Journal
CSD	Centrale des syndicats démocratiques
CSN	Confédération des syndicats nationaux
CTCC	Confédération des travailleurs catholiques du Canada
EPA	Environmental Protection Agency
FLQ	Front de libération du Québec
JM	Johns-Manville Corporation
LAC	Library and Archives Canada
PQ	Parti Québécois
QAMA	Quebec Asbestos Mining Association
SNA	Syndicat national d'Asbestos
UN	United Nations
WHO	World Health Organization
WTO	World Trade Organization

A Town Called Asbestos

Introducing Asbestos

WHAT'S IN A NAME? At the start of my research on Asbestos, Quebec, in December 2007, G. Claude Théroux of the Société d'Histoire d'Asbestos took a piece of raw asbestos from his pocket and threw it onto the table between us. "You want to know Asbestos? Now you know it."[1] Looking at the table in shock, I asked, "Aren't you afraid of getting sick?" At the start of my research, before I had begun to realize the connection the townspeople felt with asbestos, this was an understandable question. It was also a naive one. A retired history teacher who had put himself through university by working at the massive opencast Jeffrey Mine located in the centre of town, Théroux handled the mineral with a familiarity passed down to him through generations who had made Asbestos their home.

From the late nineteenth century until the 1970s, the Western world became increasingly reliant on fireproof materials made from asbestos. The town of Asbestos grew in size and influence alongside this demand. As industry increasingly added asbestos to building materials, auto parts, and household appliances, medical professionals and company officials discovered its harmful effects on human health, but they did not inform the general public or asbestos workers of the risks.

The town of Asbestos was completely dependent on this deadly industry for its survival. Because of this dependence, townspeople developed a unique, place-based understanding of their local environment, the risks they faced living next to the giant opencast asbestos mine, and their place within the global resource trade. The local–global tensions that define this history can help us understand the broad problems and possibilities other resource communities have faced, and continue to face today.

A Brief Overview

The resource town of Asbestos is located in the Eastern Townships of Quebec, Canada, halfway between Montreal and Quebec City, north of Sherbrooke and south of the St. Lawrence River (see Figure 1). It is the site of the Jeffrey Mine, once the largest opencast chrysotile asbestos mine in the world, long owned by the industry leader, the American Johns-Manville Company (JM). By examining the history of Asbestos, this book offers new perspectives on the ways in which bodies of land, human bodies, and the body politic converge in resource communities at both local and global levels.

The history of Asbestos is rooted in the mineral that lies beneath the town. The term "asbestos" encompasses six different types of the mineral found throughout the world, whose chemical makeup varies with the deposit's origins and era of formation. The white chrysotile asbestos found in places like North America, Russia, Zimbabwe, China, and Brazil was formed in serpentine rock. The five other mineral types – amosite, athophyllite, crocidolite, tremolite, and actinolite – were formed in amphibole rock.[2] Some of these possess longer fibres that are more easily woven than chrysotile, but all occur as a fibrous rock that can be broken apart by hand until it resembles raw cotton. Asbestos was added to a variety of goods to improve their resistance to burning, rust, and decay.[3] The chrysotile found in Asbestos (see Figure 2) is composed of magnesium, silicon, and oxygen ($Mg_3Si_2O_5[OH]_4$)[4] and is able to withstand temperatures in excess of 3000°F. Once considered both magical and modern because of its fireproof qualities, asbestos also causes cancer and other deadly diseases.

Although its "magical" qualities were known in the nineteenth century, the first boom in asbestos production did not occur until the First World War, when the mineral was used in soldier's uniforms and firefighting equipment. After the war, it became a key component in reconstruction efforts. International demand for asbestos was fuelled largely by society's desire for modern conveniences: fire-retardant housing materials, fireproof clothing, long-lasting cement structures, and safe and durable automobile

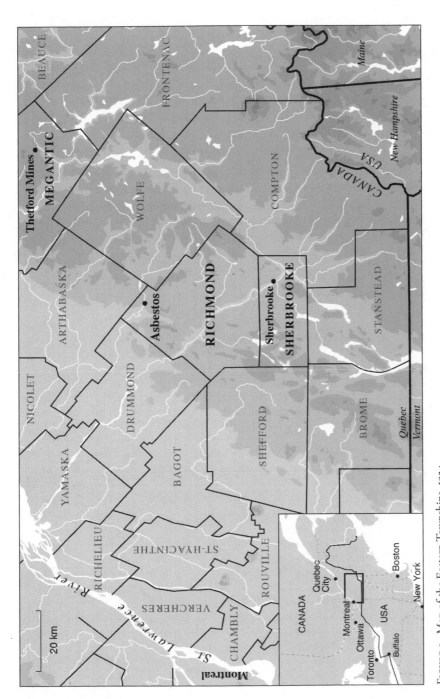

FIGURE 1 Map of the Eastern Townships, 1924
Source: Adapted from ETRC by Eric Leinberger

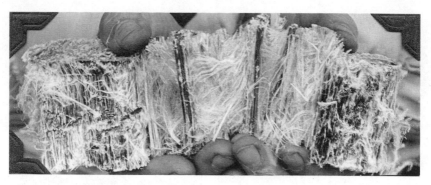

FIGURE 2   Canadian chrysotile asbestos
Source: W.G. Clark Fonds, ETRC

parts. Asbestos promised safety for those who used it and profits for those who sold it. Chrysotile asbestos from Quebec once made up 95 percent of the global trade in the mineral (see Figure 3); the Jeffrey Mine produced most of this supply.[5] To fully appreciate how these production levels influenced both land and people in Asbestos, the following chapters situate the community and its industry within a local-global framework of large-scale environmental change, contamination, and resilience during the twentieth century.

While the Jeffrey Mine remained partly active until 2012, I use 1983 – the year Johns-Manville sold the mine after declaring bankruptcy – as a key date in its history and as the end date for this study. As geographer David Robertson writes, "all mines eventually cease to be profitable ... In the majority of historic mining areas, however, remote locations and poorly diversified economies have ensured economic stagnation and decline following mine closure."[6] When I first began examining Asbestos in 2005, I considered 1983 to be the year the town collapsed, for without Johns-Manville operating the Jeffrey Mine, the town – and the industry – went into sharp, terminal decline. But as my research and study developed, I began to understand how survival and resilience play a central role in resource communities, which are so vulnerable to local and global changes.

Reading the volume *Questioning Collapse*, edited by Patricia A. McAnany and Norman Yoffee, further convinced me that survival was an important element in the history of Asbestos. McAnany and Yoffee posit that while corporations and industries may collapse, societies never do. Instead, "when closely examined, the overriding human story is one of survival

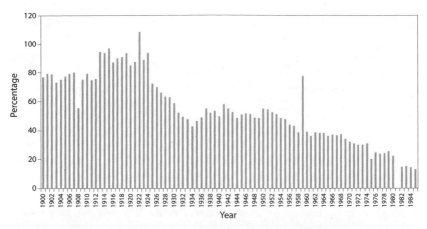

FIGURE 3 Quebec asbestos production as a percentage of world production, 1900–85

Note: There is a discrepancy in the figure for 1922, which reads as 108 percent of global supply, which is obviously incorrect, although I have found no data to suggest which number is wrong, so I have left it as is.

Source: The Quebec data is based on data provided by the Reports on Mining Operations (1898-1936) and on the Mining Industry of the Province of Quebec (1937-2000) (http://www.mern.gouv.qc.ca/mines/desminesetdeshommes/index.jsp#annexe), compiled by Marc Vallières. I have converted the short tons on the list to metric tons to more easily compare with the world data, which was provided by the United States Geological Survey, Circular 1298, Robert L. Virta, "Worldwide Asbestos Supply and Consumption Trends from 1900 through 2003, 2006 (http://pubs.usgs.gov/circ/2006/1298/c1298.pdf) 32-34.

and regeneration. Certainly crises existed, political forms changed, and landscapes were altered, but rarely did societies collapse in an absolute and apocalyptic sense."[7] This study shows that in the resource community of Asbestos, where the people and the land are so closely linked, the redefinition of the Jeffrey Mine from profitable to hazardous forced community members to adapt in order to ensure their survival.

There were other asbestos mines in the world, and other asbestos-producing companies, but for much of the twentieth century, none of them were as large or as far-reaching as the Jeffrey Mine and JM. The tons and tons of asbestos fibre that Jeffrey Mine workers extracted each day were shipped to factories around the world to be turned into household and industrial goods. This was a remarkable movement of community land, and the following chapters will highlight these changes alongside an analysis of the medical and political history of Asbestos to show how utilitarian perspectives on local environmental use influenced the global industry.

The history of Asbestos reveals local residents engaged in a constant struggle for balance between the community and the mine, while maintaining a commitment to both. This balance was affected by the interactions between the working-class French Canadian majority and the anglophone managerial elite, and between both and the natural world, and gave character and purpose to the land, the people, and the politics of Asbestos. While townspeople were often divided, their actions and reactions were rooted in their commitment to using the local environment to the fullest possible extent, and this raises questions about how the boundaries between people and the natural world dissolve in resource communities to shape a character that is unique to place.

So this book examines the local character of Asbestos and – echoing the insights of geographers Anthony C. Gatrell and Susan J. Elliott – shows that "people help to create places, and in turn people are shaped by the places they inhabit."[8] This includes how a community adapts to environmental change and contamination in order to survive. By structuring its analysis around bodies of land, human bodies, and the body politic, *Asbestos* folds together the environmental, medical, and political history of the town to show how its people understood place, self, and risk as they focused almost entirely on the success of the Jeffrey Mine, and the dangers – industrial and environmental – that residents confronted each day.

BODIES OF LAND

There were three interconnected physical realities in Asbestos: the mineral, the Jeffrey Mine, and the land on which the community was built. These I term bodies of land. The global demand for the mineral encouraged high extraction levels at the Jeffrey Mine, which periodically expanded into the community, displacing both homes and businesses.

Historical studies of land have been fundamental to the field of environmental history, in which the relationship between culture and the natural world is a key pillar. Environmental historian Richard White has urged scholars to re-examine the connection between work and nature, asserting that through labour, humans and the natural world become inseparable.[9] This book extends this idea by showing that bodily knowledge of nature is gained not only by those who work directly with it, such as the men and women at the Jeffrey Mine, but also by those who live around it. The people of Asbestos knew the land through work, but men, women, and children, young and old, also knew it intimately simply by living in the community:

hearing the sounds of the machines in the pit, seeing and breathing the asbestos dust that hovered over neighbourhoods, experiencing the terror of rocks crashing through their homes during blasting, and using the mine as a focal point of celebration, community spirit, and play. In much the same way that the rapid industrialization of British Columbia's timber industry turned the forest into a giant factory without a roof,[10] the Jeffrey Mine was a factory in the heart of the community. Johns-Manville constantly introduced new technologies to improve extraction rates and meet the rising international demand for asbestos. Far from distancing the workers from the resource they were extracting (as scholars have found occurring in other locales[11]), these new technologies and a booming global market strengthened and politicized the connection between people and the natural world.

HUMAN BODIES

Pride and risk combined to define the community of Asbestos. The following chapters show how the connection between people and land can negatively affect human bodies – those of Jeffrey Mine workers and those of members of the broader community of Asbestos – and how those affected have confronted or ignored this reality. Medical histories too often separate the disease from the body.[12] By analyzing the lived experiences of those whose health the mineral directly affected, and of those who had to reconcile the dangerous land on which they worked with the community land on which they lived, this book humanizes the three main diseases caused by asbestos: asbestosis, lung cancer, and mesothelioma.

Asbestosis results from the inhalation of microscopic asbestos fibres over an extended period. Typically, those fibres build up in and harden the lining of the lungs, preventing them from expanding and contracting as they should. This leads to death by suffocation. Lung cancer is more commonly known, but because of the disease's association with tobacco, historically, industry-funded medical professionals who examined Jeffrey Mine workers were often able to attribute their lung disease to smoking cigarettes, not asbestos exposure[13] – much to the advantage of asbestos companies. Mesothelioma is another asbestos-related cancer; it manifests itself in the linings of major organs, resulting in a fast-progressing, rarely curable disease. Skin, breast, ovary, and colon cancer are among the other diseases the mineral causes. All of these are extremely painful, can take between fifteen and thirty years to develop, and require an uncertain dose/

longevity of exposure to develop. This means, simply, that *any* exposure to asbestos can be dangerous to human health.

Rachel Carson's *Silent Spring*, published in 1962, is widely celebrated as one of the first books to elucidate the connection between human health and environmental contamination. Since then, scholars of global industries have attempted to bring large corporations that are responsible for environmental contamination to account. Matters of risk and health have historically been viewed in terms of class. People seem to expect miners to get sick, as if it is part of the job, and this plays into traditional stereotypes about working-class populations and lifestyles. This understanding has its roots in the Victorian era, when medical professionals and company officials began to regulate working-class culture through health reform.[14] For much of the history examined in the following chapters, companies, courts, unions, and the media knew that asbestos was harmful to human health, but the mineral was so important to Western society that the industry survived well beyond initial reports of public risk and disease.

All of this allowed JM to use the community of Asbestos as a perfectly contained test laboratory, with citizens unknowingly acting as lab mice. In *Asbestos*, I provide a close examination of how townspeople slowly came to know about the risks they were subject to and how they internalized this knowledge to help the community – and the Jeffrey Mine – survive.

THE BODY POLITIC

A local understanding of risk and of the connections between humans and the natural environment also defined the body politic in Asbestos. This was a community sharply divided by class into three factions: Jeffrey Mine workers; middle-class community leaders; and upper-class company officials. A rich literature on risk illuminates how the community reacted to the mineral's negative health effects. Major works by Mary Douglas and Ulrich Beck encourage us to think of risks as political entities around which societies see and shape themselves.[15] Furthermore, risk is not a stagnant or finite thing – rather, it operates on a sliding scale, with severity determined by people, place, and time. A risk that a miner deems acceptable to himself may not, even in his estimation, be acceptable for his children. The people of Asbestos were aware of the dangers the mineral posed to their bodies well before it became a public issue, but they chose to attempt to manage the risks rather than reject the industry that gave the community purpose.

The local commitment to community survival in Asbestos was articulated in lived experience. Historian Joy Parr explains this process when she writes that "bodies are not only being *conditioned* by circumstances, they are also enduring reservoirs of past practice, which *actively influence* subsequent responses."[16] So my focus on bodies in this book, and on the unconscious knowledge they can reveal, relies on Parr's concept of embodiment and distinguishes this study from other histories of mining communities. My highlighting of the women at the Jeffrey Mine and the agency the community exercised when it came to decisions on environmental development also distinguishes this study from many other mining histories.[17]

Rather than simply bowing to the will of a distant corporate headquarters, the people of Asbestos insisted again and again on keeping issues surrounding land and people local. Thus, they resented any action that breached the community's borders. This book, too, will remain mostly within the community's borders as it details a local history of this global industry. I will be arguing that land, health, and politics in this small Québécois town contributed to the asbestos industry's exponential rise, as well as its thundering collapse.

NECESSARY BOUNDARIES

This book shows that place matters when we consider the reasons for, and effects of, large-scale environmental change and contamination. Environmentally, medically, and politically, there is something unique and hitherto unexamined about Asbestos. The mine is the source of the community's pride and sorrow, success and decline, but to those from outside Asbestos, the town is widely known for two other reasons.

First, Asbestos was the scene of a dramatic strike between February and June 1949, a strike that some historians contend launched Quebec's Quiet Revolution, a socio-political movement in which the province's French Canadian majority became increasingly secular, gained control of the province's major industries and businesses, and rallied their political strength to bring about major changes in Quebec and the rest of Canada.[18] These changes – and the strike itself – were, of course, not limited to Asbestos, but by examining the tension between the working-class francophone majority and the anglophone elite who filled managerial roles at the Jeffrey Mine, this study will be examining key themes of the Quiet Revolution relevant to other resource communities in the province, such as Shawinigan and Abitibi-Témiscamingue.

The principal publication to emerge from the 1949 strike was Pierre Elliott Trudeau's edited collection, *La Grève de l'amiante*, published in 1956. In his introduction, Trudeau wrote that "it is the date, rather than the particular place or the industry that is decisive."[19] This book shows that Trudeau was wrong: the people, the place, and the industry involved in the 1949 strike were what made the dispute matter, not just in the history of Quebec but also in the history of Canada and the history of international trade and labour. Aside from a local history produced for the town's centenary in 1999, and a short article on the encroachment of the Jeffrey Mine on the town in 1967, this book is the first in-depth study of the community that focuses on more than the five-month strike of 1949, and it is the only one that examines the subject from the perspective of environmental history.

The strike was a local conflict with global ramifications because the industry had international reach and also because those involved in publicizing it became major figures in Québécois and Canadian political history. Maurice Duplessis, who often plays the villain's role in these accounts, was Quebec premier for eighteen years and had a powerful impact on the province's development. Jean Marchand, secretary for the Confédération des travailleurs catholiques du Canada (CTCC) union, slept in the homes of workers during the strike and went on to become a federal cabinet minister, a senator, and a Companion of the Order of Canada. Gérard Pelletier, a university friend of Marchand and reporter for the influential Montreal newspaper *Le Devoir*, became a federal cabinet minister, a Canadian ambassador, and a Companion of the Order of Canada. Pierre Trudeau, who briefly joined Pelletier in Asbestos, was prime minister of Canada for fifteen years. André Laurendeau and Pierre Laporte wrote for *Le Devoir* on the provincial implications of the strike and later served in the Quebec legislature.

The role of these historical figures in the 1949 strike has turned Asbestos into a place of symbol and myth regarding the state of Quebec on the eve of the Quiet Revolution. This book brings the community and the reasons for the miners' labour militancy back into the history of the strike to show how a local perspective can tell a broader history about resource towns, industrialization, health, risk, and political influence. The history of

Asbestos concerns much more than a labour dispute, and only Chapter 5 focuses on the 1949 strike, offering a play-by-play analysis of the conflict as it unfolded and irrevocably changed the community.

Second, Asbestos is widely known because from 1983 until 2012, the town received financial and political support from federal and provincial governments to keep the Jeffrey Mine, and therefore the town, alive, despite the mineral's known adverse effects on human health.[20] In other words, Canada exploited its generally positive international image to cast shadows over medical reports proving the dangers of asbestos, to avoid strict regulation of chrysotile in global markets, and to sell the mineral to developing countries, where workers and other citizens were neither adequately informed about the risks nor protected from them.

These aspects of the asbestos trade are not addressed in this study, which finds its end point in its examination of how environment, health, and politics contributed to the rise of Asbestos, followed by its decline in 1983, when Johns-Manville left the community after filing for bankruptcy the previous year. This is not to diminish the role Canada played in keeping the deadly industry alive for over thirty years after Western markets for the mineral had collapsed, and after the dangers of asbestos became widely known. With their stories of government officials making suspect alliances and continuously prioritizing industry over human health, the chapters that follow suggest that recent aspects of this story are a haunting echo of long-established patterns of behaviour.

I contend that 1983 was the end of an important era in Asbestos, marked by massive profits and corporate deceit but also by community pride. The Jeffrey Mine was the biggest of its kind in the world for much of the twentieth century, Johns-Manville was the largest asbestos-producing company during this same time period, and the community of Asbestos connected the two. By returning scholarly focus to the community of Asbestos, I hope this book offers new analysis of how environmental change, contamination, and collapse affect resource towns, emphasizing the local-global connections and tensions that industry brings to a community, and that community brings to the world.[21]

THIS BOOK IS ABOUT the interaction of bodies of land, human bodies, and the body politic. Chapter 1 traces the origins of the asbestos industry in Quebec, the opening of the Jeffrey Mine, and the founding of the town by examining geological shifts, human migration, and the development of a community reliant on a single resource. It shows how these elements interacted in Asbestos before the First World War, during which New York's H.W. Johns-Manville Co. purchased the Jeffrey Mine and thereby changed the character of the community.

Chapter 2 is the first of three focusing on the 1918–49 period between the arrival of JM in Asbestos and the strike of 1949. In this chapter, I focus on the changes JM made in Asbestos by expanding the boundaries of the mine, introducing new technologies for industrial efficiency, and convincing local residents that production came before people and that residents needed to make sacrifices for the community's survival.

Chapter 3 examines environmental contamination and health between the wars. It relies on confidential medical reports detailing the spread of asbestos-related disease in the community and shows how JM prevented this knowledge from reaching workers and the general public. It also situates Asbestos within historical literature on industrial health and hazards[22] and examines how JM gained power over medical evidence – and the bodies of their workers – by allying itself with medical researchers and insurance companies to present the most benign view possible of the risks asbestos posed to human health.

One of the most fascinating aspects of the community of Asbestos is its commitment to the Jeffrey Mine despite the risks associated with it. In Chapter 4, we see that this commitment was linked to a sense of ownership. JM was powerful, but the people of Asbestos demonstrated their autonomy through strikes and protests whenever they saw the company developing the Jeffrey Mine in ways with which they disagreed. This chapter also illustrates the agency of community members despite the constraints that come with living in a single-resource, single-company town, and shows how invested they were in the changes that benefited or threatened their survival.

Labour historians have long viewed the 1949 strike in Asbestos as a turning point in the history of the working class in Canada and of the Quiet Revolution in Quebec. By focusing on land, health, and community during the conflict, Chapter 5 examines the strike as a turning point, but a profoundly local one, rooted in issues of land use, environmental health, and power. This chapter examines how the conflict changed the local population's understanding of themselves and the land.

Again pulling apart the historical perspectives in Asbestos, Chapter 6 focuses on how land was used, changed, and understood in the community between the 1949 strike and 1983, when JM sold the Jeffrey Mine. It provides an in-depth analysis of large-scale landscape change as production levels increased at the Jeffrey Mine and as the community surrounding it made physical and ideological sacrifices to facilitate the industrial transformation of the environment.

In Chapter 7, I examine how growing public awareness of asbestos-related disease affected Jeffrey Mine workers and other members of the community. As the industry rapidly declined around them, Jeffrey Mine workers became its biggest advocates, minimizing the risks it posed and using their own bodies to show they were unaffected by asbestos-related disease. Much of this was based on the false information about the mineral's effects that JM had provided its employees for decades, but it also reveals significant working-class agency in Asbestos. Jeffrey Mine workers were increasingly exposed to reports that proved asbestos was dangerous to them and the general public, but as the industry collapsed, many of them chose to diminish the risks and their own bodily knowledge for the sake of community survival.

In the final chapter, I examine how local residents negotiated the challenges generated by the industry's decline between 1949 and 1983. Through an analysis of local, national, and international efforts to keep the Jeffrey Mine open and the population of Asbestos employed in the late 1970s and early 1980s, I show both the vulnerability and the resilience of resource communities confronting industrial collapse and environmental contamination. How townspeople dealt with this physical reality was directly informed by their history over this time period.

Each of these chapters begins with a brief look at Asbestos today, to show how the past is reflected in the present. As a whole, this book offers a chronological examination of the ways environmental change, contamination, and resilience have added texture and depth to the histories of Asbestos and the global asbestos trade. This book explores the blurring of the boundaries between humans and the natural environment and highlights the local-global relationship between resource industries and international trade networks. Along the way, it illustrates how radical landscape change and environmental risk collided in Asbestos; it also broadens our understanding of how resource communities negotiate and accept risk by creating place-based definitions of health and survival.

Through cyclical booms and busts, "asbestos" became not simply what the local population mined or where they were, but a commitment to place, people, and community. In the process of working the Jeffrey Mine and establishing a community around it, the people of Asbestos entered into a relationship of mutual exchange with the land, shaping it and being shaped by it. How does a community take shape around a constantly growing open pit mine? How do communities develop a local understanding of health? Who defines risk and danger, and how? Can a small resource community influence global trade policy? How do international borders and networks complicate local self-determination? This book answers these questions as it examines the history of the Jeffrey Mine and the community that surrounded it.

I

Creation Stories: Asbestos before 1918

THE APPALACHIAN MOUNTAINS surrounding the community of Asbestos act as a striking balance point to the opencast Jeffrey Mine, which is located in the centre of town. Indeed, it is difficult to avoid either as you walk the streets of the community today, especially once you realize that both were created by the same geological shifts and collisions millions of years ago. Asbestos fibre was born of geological friction and heat. Asbestos the place would follow suit, being created and re-created with the friction and heat of clashing cultures, ideologies, and aspirations. The asbestos deposits of southeastern Quebec were shaped by the breakup of the hypothesized supercontinent Rodinia at the beginning of the Precambrian period 750 million years ago. Major tectonic shifts pushed mountain chains that were once part of the ocean floor into the land mass that was to become North America during the Devonian period between 410 and 355 million years ago, creating the Appalachian Mountains, a range extending from Greenland to the southern United States, passing through what was to become Asbestos. The intense heat and friction of this process chemically reconstituted the serpentine rock at this particular site, and in its recrystallization, the chemical composition was changed and veins of asbestos fibre were formed.[1]

The Jeffrey Mine resulted from a geological quirk. Most of the world's asbestos is found in veins, usually several metres in length, arrayed along a linear plane. This meant that a number of mines were often established beside one another to access entire deposits. By contrast, the asbestos deposit near the town of that name was found in circular veins forming a rounded knoll of marketable asbestos. This deposit could be exploited, in its entirety, by opencast extraction at a single pit that became the Jeffrey Mine.

Scientific interest in the geology of this area began with the founding of the Canadian Geological Survey (CGS) in 1842. William Edmond Logan, a British-educated Montrealer and the first head of the survey,[2] was fascinated by the geological past of the region. In his first survey report on Quebec, he offered a detailed description of the area that would become Asbestos. Fellow surveyor Alexander Murray also examined the geological history of the region, searching for rocks and minerals of economic value. Noting the presence of green serpentine rock that would be excellent for ornamental architecture, Murray wrote that it would be of value only "when free from veins of asbestus [sic]."[3] The mineral had little practical application and no economic value.

The GSC was pessimistic about the region's agricultural prospects. Even so, the colonial government built railways through the region, which led to dramatic social, economic, and environmental change. With the opening of the Grand Trunk Railway in 1852, people flocked to the region to settle and farm along the line, which bypassed the future site of Asbestos by four miles. At the time, other parts of Lower Canada were facing a population crisis. By 1862, the Eastern Townships had a population of 200,000, largely due to the influx of French Canadians.

In the 1870s, workers constructing the Quebec Central Railway, which ran through the Eastern Townships on its way from Lake Huron to Quebec City, uncovered significant amounts of asbestos near the community of Thetford. The discovery came at an opportune time, for American manufacturers were starting to specialize in asbestos-based building products to meet a growing demand in the industrializing United States.[4] As the nineteenth century ended, different factions of the Eastern Townships' population – English, French, upper class, working class – fought over who controlled the land. Asbestos was often central to this struggle.

For many years, geologists and industry experts had considered the deposits at Thetford, 100 kilometres from Asbestos, to be the largest in the world. Industry leaders and workers looking for employment soon came to know this area as the "asbestos belt."[5] Because of the CGS's detailed descriptions of the region, the mineral was easily identifiable to those without geological training. This was how gentleman farmer William H. Jeffrey discovered the mineral in the late 1870s. He convinced Charles Webb, who owned the land, to go into business with him. It is not clear how the two met, nor is it clear how exactly Jeffrey discovered the asbestos deposit on Webb's land. However, once the discovery had been made, Jeffrey controlled the mine operations and Webb controlled the budget. While neither knew the full extent of the deposit, Jeffrey and Webb's efforts in 1879 began a major redefinition of the land on which they would help establish the town of Asbestos.

AN ENVIRONMENTAL REVOLUTION, 1879–99

A year after Jeffrey's discovery of asbestos, the Acte général des mines du Québec established new mining regulations to ensure that the government received a portion of any profits that came from the land.[6] In 1881, the year in which the Quebec government appointed Joseph Obalski as director of mining services, Jeffrey and Webb employed fourteen men – seven French Canadians and seven English Canadians – to clear the land and begin mining asbestos.[7] The work was slow and arduous.

Carving out the opencast Jeffrey Mine involved a real physical struggle with the land. Operations only took place in the summer, when the earth was neither frozen by the cold nor flooded by the thaw.[8] A crew would clear the surface soil with picks, shovels, and the occasional ox-driven scraping cart until they uncovered the bottle-green serpentine rock, which contained veins of asbestos between five and twenty feet down. Workers would then blast free large pieces of rock surrounded by asbestos veins.[9] They would then bring the chunks of rock to the cobbing shop, where boys broke it apart with hammers and sorted the asbestos fibres according to length.[10]

The dangers involved in blasting large rocks out of the ground meant that the population growing around the Jeffrey Mine understood physical risk.[11] Health care was not a primary concern for the workers carving out the Jeffrey Mine, and regional access to doctors was limited. Miners had to accept the risks that came with their occupation; if they were injured, there was a chance they would die. The biggest health threat associated with asbestos at this time was the act of mining itself; there was no awareness of the specific dangers asbestos posed to human health.

In the nineteenth century, the medical profession in Quebec was deeply divided along linguistic lines. The province was the first in Canada to form a regulated medical society, but until 1843, McGill University was the only institution in Quebec allowed to grant medical degrees, and it did so only in English.[12] The Association des médecins de langue française de l'Amérique du Nord, established in 1902, oriented itself towards the

medical community in France, not North America, and because the
Catholic Church was responsible for establishing and running hospitals
and clinics in Quebec, medical knowledge was often overpowered by religious ideology.

Besides being dangerous, extracting fibre from the Jeffrey Mine was
time-consuming. Because market prices for asbestos were based on fibre
length – with the longest being the most valuable – opencast mining
provided the best access to full veins of the mineral. It also had a tremendous ecological impact on the land. In 1880s Canada, opencast mining
had strong, practical advantages over underground. Engineer Fritz Cirkel
explained to the Canadian Department of Mines that opencast pits allowed
for easier supervision, made total extraction of the asbestos fibre possible
due to the lack of underground structural pillars, and provided clean air
for workers to breathe.[13] The disadvantages of opencast mining, Cirkel
explained, were that it was difficult to remove barren serpentine rock,
operations were often halted because of poor weather, and there was a
limited amount of space where waste rock and fibre could be dumped.
Because of the amount of surrounding farmland available to them, Jeffrey
and Webb committed to the opencast method, and a community grew
around the expanding pit. All of this shaped how the local population
understood themselves and their local environment.

By 1884, a post office had been built close to the Jeffrey-Webb mine
with a sign on the front of it reading "Asbestos."[14] The fact that a government agency gave the community an English name rather than the French
equivalent, "amiante," suggests the extent to which anglophone landownership and connections dominated the increasingly francophone region. This was certainly the case at the anglophone-run Jeffrey Mine, which
by 1886 the CGS described as "a mine of considerable extent [that] has
been operated for several years ... This industry has already grown to large
proportions, and bids fair to become one of the most important in the
Dominion."[15] Surveyors and prospectors in the 1880s scoured the region
for untapped asbestos deposits with which to earn their fortunes, as it
seemed Jeffrey and Webb had.

The Jeffrey Mine was thriving, and went from employing fourteen men
working only during the summer months in 1881, to seventy men working
all seasons and extracting fifteen tons of the mineral each week in 1885.[16]
This created a less transient community at Asbestos than was common in
the region's other resource towns. The miners' families, who once lived four
miles away in Danville, slowly moved to Asbestos as the community took
shape near the mine. Fifteen tons a week was enough to ensure that the

Jeffrey Mine – and the community growing around it – was economically viable, but that amount paled by comparison to the extraction levels at the mines near Thetford, where the real asbestos fever was centred. According to the CGS, in 1885 the four mines at Thetford employed 250 men at "the largest and most important operations" in the region and extracted 1,100 tons during the summer months alone.[17] The Jeffrey Mine was decidedly second-rate in comparison and was often referred to as "the small mine near Danville" long after Asbestos was incorporated as a village in 1899.

Enthusiastic about the riches its borders contained, Canada showcased the Dominion's natural resources, including asbestos, at the 1886 Colonial and Indian Exhibition in London, England. Referring to the Thetford display, the official report noted that there was great interest in the industry, and several mines were sold during the event.[18] This was a positive reception, but the properties sold were far from Asbestos, and surveyors believed that although the Jeffrey Mine's output was considerable, it was also limited. The true value of the deposit at Asbestos had yet to be discovered.

The Jeffrey Mine contained veins of asbestos that were much smaller than those at Thetford, and those veins were strangely broken up throughout the deposit. This resulted in shorter, less valuable fibres. Because the value of asbestos in the late nineteenth century was based on fibre length (longer fibres meant quicker processing and spinning into a wool-like yarn), Thetford's mineral was more desirable. Furthermore, the area surrounding the Jeffrey Mine was still being used for farming, which restricted the industry's expansion even as land ripe for industrialization was being purchased elsewhere at $5 an acre.[19] Because of these constraints, the CGS stressed that "there is no apparent reason why [asbestos] should not be found in paying quantity at other points, and it is possible that subsequent exploration will largely extend the area where profitable mining operations can be carried on."[20]

Quebec's Director of Mines was equally optimistic. Since his appointment in 1881, Joseph Obalski had been visiting mines throughout Quebec and promoting the province's minerals on the international markets. Because Obalski was an engineer and not a geologist, his publications differed somewhat from those of the CGS, though they shared an overall excitement about the asbestos industry, which extracted 6,000 tons of fibre in 1889.[21] The Jeffrey Mine contributed 207 tons to this total, and 400 tons the following year, but these were insignificant figures compared to those coming from Thetford, which mined 4,803 tons in 1890.[22]

The increase in the amount of asbestos extracted by miners in the Eastern Townships fuelled Obalski's excitement over the industry's importance to the economic future of Quebec. He wrote that the people of the region produced more asbestos than anywhere else in the world, because of the abundance of the mineral and the region's sophisticated transportation network. He also expressed his enthusiasm for the industry: a "remarkable fact ... is that, while the production has increased with the demand, prices have also risen, so that, of late years, asbestos lands have been eagerly sought after. This is owing to the new uses which are being daily discovered."[23] Rising prices and demand for asbestos led to an increase in the number of prospectors in the region, who hoped to take advantage of the land and the market.

The Jeffrey Mine was profitable, but by 1887 ambition had exceeded ability. Jeffrey cut back the number of men he employed at the pit. The industry had stagnated in Quebec, partly because it focused only on extracting the raw mineral, which workers then packaged and sent to the more industrialized United States or Great Britain for further processing. This limited the type of employment and extent of returns in the mining communities of the region. Mine owners and government officials were not interested in what happened to the asbestos after workers extracted it, and CGS geologists constantly urged the development of more asbestos pits, not processing plants. Plans to industrialize the region focused on natural resources in their raw form. Factories did not yet figure into how people saw and used the land. With a clear focus on mining the raw mineral, engineers in the region's asbestos industry developed new extraction technologies to boost the amount of rock being taken from the mines.[24]

The first mechanization of the industry came in the late 1880s with the introduction of compressed air and steam power for drilling blasting holes and hoisting ore in Thetford. This new technology helped the mines there thrive. Meanwhile, production at the Jeffrey Mine dwindled. When Obalski visited in 1889, he noted that the pit, which contained mostly short fibre, was roughly 100 feet deep and located on the plateau of a knoll about 180 feet above the surrounding area. The thirty-five workers at the mine did not use any mechanized technology, and they no longer worked in the winter.[25] In 1885, Jeffrey and Webb had employed seventy men, who had extracted over 700 tons of asbestos annually by working yearlong. Four years later, operations had not advanced technologically and production had declined to 325 tons annually. Half the workforce had moved on, transportation costs from Asbestos to the Grand Trunk were high, and the mine was poorly managed.

Neither Jeffrey nor Webb was an engineer or a geologist, and their understanding of the land at Asbestos was rudimentary. Their lack of knowledge was indicative of an industry-wide misunderstanding of the deposit. In his 1897 book on global asbestos deposits, British geologist Robert H. Jones described Jeffrey and Webb:

> It must not be supposed, that [their] want of knowledge was in any way blameable, because if this were so, then it must be said that all those commercial and scientific men who had, year after year, examined the property, or viewed it mineralogically, were equally so. Nothing of the peculiar nature and quality of the serpentine in which [they] worked was then known.[26]

Those who ran the Jeffrey Mine – and the surveyors and engineers who studied it – did not yet understand the uniqueness of the land at Asbestos.

Despite the dwindling fortunes of the Jeffrey Mine, and of others, surveyors and prospectors continued to search the region for profitable asbestos deposits. The Canadian economy suffered a depression from 1873 to 1896, and the Dominion had only its natural resources on which to rely. Seeing an opportunity, in 1887 the CGS stressed that key regions needed to be surveyed again to reassess the value of the resources found there, especially asbestos.[27] Although some mines were failing, the rising value of the mineral in international markets drew prospectors back to the Eastern Townships for another look. The result was an asbestos rush that left many financially ruined and the land torn apart.

Obalski urged caution to those in search of asbestos, noting that the presence of serpentine rock did not automatically mean the mineral would be found nearby,[28] but prospectors continued to dig up the land near serpentine outcroppings in the hope of finding the valuable fibre. Failed mines soon scarred the region's landscape. In 1892, American asbestos manufacturing companies amalgamated as the H.W. Johns Manufacturing Co. and began scouring the region for a viable mine that could feed its operations. The company did not hone in on the Jeffrey Mine at this time, because, just a year after *Canadian Mining and Mechanical Review* had described it as "one of the best" producers of asbestos, the Jeffrey Mine went bankrupt.[29] Mere months before this, a visiting reporter had described "between 600 and 700 people, all dependent on the mine," in Asbestos, where two farmhouses and a small school had stood only six years before.[30]

One reason for the failure of the Jeffrey Mine was its owners. Webb took a backseat in the business, while Jeffrey was not well connected in the industry and chose not to belong to the Asbestos Club, an association of the region's mine owners who met monthly to discuss new technologies

and forge new connections. The Asbestos Club was an important factor
in the success of the Thetford mines because it facilitated the exchange
of knowledge and extraction techniques. It also created a strong community identity among local miners, regardless of the company they worked
for. Isolated by distance and by Jeffrey's character – he was described as
"somewhat obstinate and self-willed, and strictly a man of the old school
– independent in his ideas, by no means highly educated, and never
much inclined to move out of the old grooves"[31] – the mine at Asbestos
languished.

The four-and-a-half to five tons of asbestos extracted daily from Jeffrey's
mine failed to meet the $4,000 monthly payroll.[32] When Jeffrey and
Webb went bankrupt, people quickly left Asbestos. The locals became part
of the region's transient workforce, flocking to new pits when they opened,
then retreating back to the more stable mines at Thetford when they closed,
with families being left behind during periods of instability. As new resource
extraction ventures increasingly industrialized the land, worker transiency
became widespread and industries rose and fell according to market
demand.

Mine closures were common in late-nineteenth-century Quebec. Many
industry leaders blamed these failures on the provincial government's
management of the land.[33] According to Honoré Mercier, premier from
1887 to 1891, provincial revenue belonged to the francophone population,
not to the anglophone colonizers who controlled industrial development.
The success of the province was rooted in its ability to do what it wished
with its natural resources and reap the resulting profits. Implementing what
Canadian Mining and Mechanical Review deemed a "race and revenge"
style of governing, in 1890, Mercier imposed a 3 percent tax on the output
of Quebec mines and mandated the repossession of mining land that had
lain idle for more than two years. This was widely unpopular with industry leaders, who believed it would "convert the Quebec mining men
into straight anarchists,"[34] and the bill was repealed under the new government in 1892.

Despite the government's attempts to change land and resource management in Quebec, the Jeffrey Mine did not remain closed for long. In 1893
the neighbouring Danville Slate Co. bought the seventy-five acres of land
given up by Jeffrey and Webb. Industry reports indicated that this "property
is one of exceptional value, and will be exploited vigorously."[35] A new
workforce of young French Canadians drawn from the overcrowded farms
of their fathers came to Asbestos as operations resumed.

French Canadians soon came to dominate the workforce, and the new manager, Feodor Boas, understood the land quite differently than Jeffrey, Webb, or any of the engineers and geologists who had previously studied the deposit. British geologist Robert H. Jones wrote that Boas was "not an asbestos man, nor did he make any pretence to a knowledge of mineralogy, but all throughout the province he was highly esteemed for his uprightness, shrewdness, and sound common sense."[36] His way of looking at the land created an asbestos revolution in the community.

Along with the pit, the Danville Slate Co purchased all the waste rock that had been taken from the mine over the previous fifteen years. Jeffrey had considered this to be useless rock that hindered the mine's success, but Boas saw it as the source of its future wealth. He discovered what Jeffrey had not: the piles of waste that workers had taken from the Jeffrey Mine since 1881 were actually piles of asbestic: asbestos fibres that industry experts thought had little value because they were too short to be woven.[37] The presence of asbestic was one reason why Jeffrey, who prided himself on his strict grading system while being unaware of the wealth he was discarding, struggled, and why geologists did not believe the mine was as valuable as the pits around Thetford.

Although asbestic could not be woven into cloth, it could be added to lead paint to fireproof walls and applied to roofing shingles to contain fires in urban areas. The once paltry demand for asbestic had risen so much in international markets by the time Boas discovered it in Asbestos that for years he had the workforce focus exclusively on the piles of waste that surrounded the pit. Boas found that once the surface rock was removed, up to 90 percent of the Jeffrey Mine was long asbestos fibres surrounded by asbestic.[38] This meant that most of what was being taken from the pit could be sold with little waste. This transformed the land into a place of extraordinary value, surpassing that of the deposits at Thetford.

Because of the demand for asbestic, employment at the Jeffrey Mine grew and old employees mixed with new as the population of Asbestos doubled in size. During Boas's first year in Asbestos, he employed 150 men; by 1895, he had increased this workforce to 400.[39] The village became home to 1,100 people, and a chapel was built to accommodate the growing community. As other mines in the region failed, the Jeffrey Mine's success increased exponentially.

The discovery of asbestic at the Jeffrey Mine coincided with a boom in the market for the product, and with a "golden age of capitalism" in Quebec based on the rapid growth of industries that exploited the province's natural

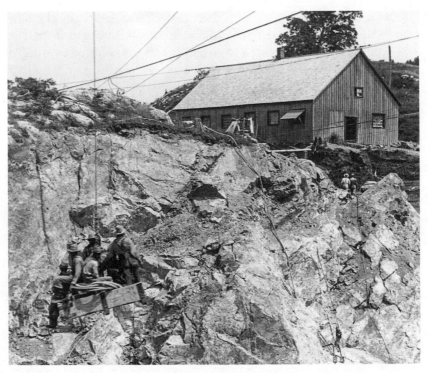

FIGURE 4   Jeffrey Mine workers being lifted out of the pit by derrick cables, 1890
Source: WG Clark Fonds, ETRC

resources.[40] This growth was international in reach, with companies from around the Western world buying into new industries. These changes could all be seen at the Jeffrey Mine, which quickly grew to become the most profitable asbestos mine in the province (see Figure 4). According to Jones,

> this mine never till now attained any special significance, [but] it has sud-denly sprung into great importance, attaining also considerable scientific interest ... In the shortest possible space of time, it has stepped in front of all the other mines previously named, and effectually [sic] revolutionized the whole asbestos industry, by bringing the use of the important mineral it deals with within the reach of the whole world. Many very important mines throughout the district are in consequence of the discoveries here, now closed.[41]

By 1896, the Jeffrey Mine was the province's leading producer of asbestos.

The dramatic increase in both population and production in Asbestos at the end of the nineteenth century altered the community and how people understood it. As the community took root, the revitalized local population built stores, churches, and blocks of new homes. No one believed that this mining town would go bust again.

To help ensure this, Boas continued his efforts to make the mine profitable. In 1896 he applied for a US patent for his invention of asbestic wall plaster. He found that when mixed with quicklime, asbestic forms a plaster that "is fireproof to the highest degree and will not crack or curl under the action of heat ... It is also ... a bad conductor of sound. As it is stronger than any other plaster, it is not necessary to have as thick a coating applied as usual, and additional economy, with a reduction of weight on the building, result."[42] Boas's asbestic plaster helped revolutionize the building industry at the turn of the twentieth century; hospitals, schools, and homes were soon coated with the fireproof, soundproof, long-lasting mineral.

Boas stressed the economic benefits of his invention: "This waste material accumulates at the mines and around the factories, and is a trouble and expense to the industry. Many attempts have been made to utilize this waste, but previous to my invention without success. My invention therefore provides a useful outlet for this waste material."[43] Overseas contracts committed the Jeffrey Mine to extracting 5,000 tons of fibre a year. New uses Boas found for the mine's output complemented other innovations and assured community members that they had a prosperous future. Those new uses also increased the value of the Jeffrey Mine, and the British Asbestos and Asbestic Co. purchased it from its local owners, bringing the mine's output to a much larger market. During the late nineteenth century, many British manufacturing companies were investing heavily in asbestos mines in places like Canada and South Africa, and the change in ownership at the Jeffrey Mine was in line with this trend. A company-built rail line connected the pit to the Grand Trunk in 1897 and further confirmed the stability of the town for the three hundred employees and their families who had made Asbestos their home.[44]

The rise in the use of electricity in industry and in urban centres at the end of the nineteenth century further boosted the Jeffrey Mine's prosperity. Fireproof insulation made of short asbestic fibres, combined with a layer of Boas's asbestic wall plaster, specifically targeted the problem of urban fires. Electricity and asbestos, both readily available in Quebec due in part to the burgeoning hydroelectricity industry, grew rapidly side by side as asbestos insulation was used around wires and in walls. This helped turn Asbestos from a transient mining camp into a permanent community,

marked by the construction of a five-storey, electrified mill for processing
the fibre post-extraction.[45] The community was incorporated as a village
of seven hundred acres in 1899, largely due to the stability Boas had brought
to the mine.

RAPID GROWTH, 1900–18

The turn of the century brought change to Asbestos as the mineral gradually became an industrial necessity and international demand rose dramatically.[46] New York's H.W. Johns-Manville Co. began to establish firm
links with the British Asbestos and Asbestic Co. and the Jeffrey Mine. The
company was formed in 1901 when New York's H.W. Johns Manufacturing Co. merged with Wisconsin's Manville Covering Co. under the
name Johns-Manville (JM).[47] Both firms specialized in manufacturing
products for the construction industry; H.W. Johns was already a leading
producer of asbestos-based products. The company had previously purchased property near Thetford that proved to be of little value, and it was
looking for a mine that would guarantee its factories a steady supply of
the mineral. One of the new company's first initiatives, in 1901, was to
purchase a controlling share of the Asbestos and Asbestic Co., which owned
the Jeffrey Mine. By 1898, most of the fibre Jeffrey Mine workers extracted
was going directly to JM in the United States for processing. By this point,
the United States was the leading manufacturer of asbestos-based goods.[48]

Closer ties to the American industry meant that the Jeffrey Mine grew
rapidly early in the twentieth century, and the village grew in tandem with
it. By 1905, Asbestos was a town of 10,000 and its output was valued at
$2,162,528. The mine's rectangular pit was now 1,200 feet long, 175 feet
wide, and 175 feet deep. This configuration exposed a variety of zones
and allowed multiple crews to access the fibre at the same time.[49] Close
to 80 percent of what workers extracted could be sold.[50] The Jeffrey Mine
became renowned for its production levels at a time when asbestos mining
was the most profitable industry in Quebec and the Eastern Townships
provided 80 percent of the world's supply.

The town of Asbestos underwent constant change during these years of
heightened production levels. No longer a mere mining camp, by 1908
the community had electricity, telephone lines, an impressive 35,000 feet
of wooden sidewalks, and new homes suitable for large families. These
were all signs of a growing, permanent community that had no fear of a
potential downturn in the industry: asbestos – and Asbestos – were here

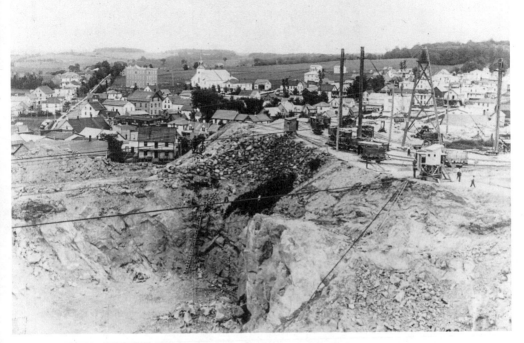

FIGURE 5   The Jeffrey Mine and the town of Asbestos, Quebec, 1909
Source: ETRC Photo Collection, ETRC

to stay. The town council pledged to do everything in its power to facilitate continued industry growth, and declared its intention to help make the "Village of Asbestos a prosperous centre that will become the City of Asbestos, and the open pit, the largest asbestos mine in the world."[51]

By 1909, the Jeffrey Mine comprised a series of eight- to fifteen-foot-high benches cut into the sides of the pit, which were worked on by several crews twenty-four hours a day.[52] The mine was rapidly becoming a giant open-air factory, and its workers were essential tools in the industrialization of the land (see Figure 5). The newly structured pit and vast mineral deposits carried output above the $2,500,000 per year mark.[53] According to the *Sherbrooke Daily Record*, the area's leading newspaper, asbestos was "king," more important than gold and silver, and the mineral from the Jeffrey Mine was of the highest quality.[54]

The industry's impressive revenues and reputation contributed to changes in government environmental policy at the beginning of the twentieth century. In the nineteenth century, Quebec had sold resource rights to private companies, with asbestos prospectors buying land for two to three dollars an acre.[55] The provincial government had also imposed a maximum 3 percent tax on the market value of any mineral extracted in Quebec. However, the increase in mining activities throughout the province led the government to increase its price for land; further payments were then required for such things as exploration permits, miner certificates, and royalties. In this way, the government generated considerable revenue. Despite these changes, the British Asbestos and Asbestic Co.'s profits continued to soar, largely because of its increasingly close relationship with JM, which seemingly had an insatiable appetite for the mineral.

The industry was booming, but wages were not. Companies were able to keep wages low because the labour supply was abundant, especially in the asbestos industry.[56] In 1912, in response to this discrepancy, thirty-six workers at Asbestos joined six hundred other provincial miners on a weeklong strike for higher wages and job security. On average, miners in the province made $1.50 to $1.75 a week, up from $1.00 between 1883 and 1900 and $1.25–$1.50 between 1900 and 1905. Unskilled workers at the Jeffrey Mine earned $1.10–$1.60 a week depending on gender, seniority, and job duties.[57] With their numbers growing from 750 in 1897 to 2,909 in 1913, Jeffrey Mine workers chose not to align with a union, fearing that labour collectives would destabilize the industry.[58] This anti-union attitude was strong throughout the province, but especially in the asbestos industry, which was known internationally for having rich mineral deposits that contributed 82 percent of the global supply, as well as for a docile working class.[59]

The demand for asbestos generated by the First World War had a significant impact on the Jeffrey Mine, the people who worked it, and the community around it. Prosperity brought major changes: the road to Danville was paved, and the first cement sidewalks were poured. The town also established a new and larger cemetery and relocated 431 coffins from the original site, partly to free it up for mine expansion.[60] Moving the cemetery was not a pleasant task, but it was one the community was willing to undertake if it meant giving the industry room to grow.

At the outbreak of the First World War, the *Canadian Mining Journal* acknowledged the importance of the mineral when it reported that "the marked increase in disastrous fires is directing more attention every day to the need of fireproof building materials that can be relied upon."[61] Canadian production rose to 139,751 short tons in 1916, worth $5,211,157. That same year, JM purchased the Jeffrey Mine fully from the Asbestos

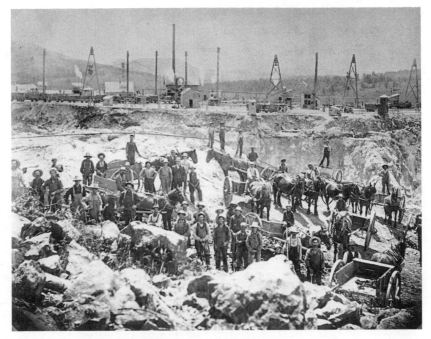

Figure 6   Stripping the land at the Jeffrey Mine, 1905
Source: WG Clark Fonds, ETRC

and Asbestic Co. Having combined mining with manufacturing, the company quickly become one of the world's leading asbestos firms. JM modernized operations at the Jeffrey Mine, where workers had long been loading raw asbestos by hand into horse-drawn dumpcarts.[62]

The Asbestos and Asbestic Co. had installed twenty-one derricks around the open pit. These tall, mast-like structures anchored a pulley system that hauled four- by six-foot train carriage boxes full of men and mineral out of the mine (see Figure 6). By 1918, JM had introduced steam shovels and a new railway line running from the bottom of the pit to the Grand Trunk at Danville, making derricks obsolete.[63]

With wartime technological advances, the company turned the Jeffrey Mine into a modern and efficient enterprise. In 1918, the *Canadian Mining Journal* reported that "now the architect, builder, steam-fitter and electrician recognize asbestos as a splendid material for resisting weather, fire, acids and other agencies of destruction, and they use it for very many purposes. The variety of uses is fast increasing and scarcely a month passes without some new application being found ... Now it is a necessary article of commerce."[64] JM was technologically advanced, economically connected, and cutthroat in its management style. The international aspirations, ideology, and reach of the company reshaped the land, the people, and the community of Asbestos.

2

Land with a Future, Not a Past,
1918–49

IN JUNE 2010, THE TOWN of Asbestos was featured on an Australian advertising show, *The Gruen Transfer*. The program's host challenged two advertising executives to create an ad campaign promoting the community. On hearing the challenge, the audience immediately began to laugh, and continued to do so as the executives talked about how difficult it was to put a positive spin on a town named Asbestos. One of the two contestants admitted that he could not get past the name, so instead he created a television commercial promoting Asbestos by highlighting other communities around the world with off-putting names, such as Accident, Maryland, and Boring, Oregon. The tag line for the commercial was, "Don't let our name put you off. Asbestos: Bad Name, Great Destination." The other ad executive attempted to use the community's name to its advantage and made a commercial called "Speed Date a Town." Competing with cities like New York and Rome, represented by suave men in expensive suits, the humble Asbestos man, dressed in a beige windbreaker, finds no dating success until the narrator says, "Great relationships are built on truth, and the truth is, we don't have a very attractive name. So spend some time online with us first, and you'll see what makes people like you fall in love with a town like us." The commercial ends with the man from Asbestos meeting his perfect match: a woman wearing a gas mask.[1]

When JM purchased the Jeffrey Mine fully in 1916, a town called Asbestos was not a bad thing. In fact, it served as a marker for the potential industrial success the resource there could give the company. JM radically transformed the land in Asbestos and how the community was connected to it. By working the Jeffrey Mine and living in such close proximity to it, the people of Asbestos developed a complex connection to the mineral and the pit, a connection facilitated by the American company's commitment to rapid growth and industrialization.

Between 1918 and 1949, JM and the people of Asbestos negotiated a balance between livable space and workable space, with the Jeffrey Mine dividing and defining the two. The community stood atop a massive asbestos deposit, and the mine that JM took over during the First World War had exposed only a small fraction of the land's wealth. From this point on, the town of Asbestos, its people, and their political priorities were forced to accommodate the increasing economic and cultural importance of the land, as well as the power of the company. Based in New York City, JM executives embraced a "bigger is better" philosophy when it came to industrial development, and the rapid growth of the Jeffrey Mine brought about by their money and technology had a tremendous impact on both the land and the community. The few local objections to this growth went unheeded as the people of Asbestos found themselves confronted time and again by the need to sacrifice the community to the mine.

SMALL SACRIFICES, 1918–23

JM was primarily an asbestos manufacturer. The company relied heavily on the Jeffrey Mine to supply its factories, processing plants, and customers. It opened its first Canadian Johns-Manville (C-JM) branch in Montreal so that top executives would be closer to the operations. As it did so, it significantly expanded the infrastructure at the mine, as needed for resource extraction. It also paid the government a substantial amount in taxes. In the postwar period, the international demand for many of Quebec's minerals boomed, and the province amended its Loi des mines so as to increase the maximum tax on extracted ore from 3 percent to 5 percent, and the minimum from 2 percent to 3.5 percent in 1916, and 5 percent in 1920 (see Figure 7).[2]

The land at Asbestos was an inverted mountain of marketable product. As JM increased extraction levels in order to access more product, it also increased its mine workforce and the hours they worked. Each day at noon and 5:30 p.m., activity in Asbestos came to a halt as the sound of blasting dynamite came from the pit, marking the turnover of each shift.[3]

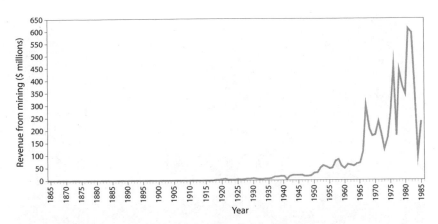

FIGURE 7   Quebec government revenue from mining pursuits, 1864-1985

Notes: The period between 1864-1921 begins with 30 June as the financial year; the period 1921-61 begins with either 30 June or 31 March as the financial year; and the period 1961-2011 begins with 31 March as the financial year.

Source: Data provided by the Province of Quebec (1937-2000) (http://www.mern.gouv.qc.ca/mines/desminesetdeshommes/index.jsp#annexe), compiled by Marc Vallières

In May 1918, JM requested permission from the Asbestos town council to run a railway line across rue St-Georges, one of the principal streets of the town.[4] The council granted permission for the railway but reserved the right to change the rail line in two years if it hindered the community in any way. In the two trial years that followed, council and most towns-people subscribed to JM's way of looking at the town's land. The success of Asbestos was quickly and firmly linked to the mine, and town council rooted many of its decisions in what JM wanted, not necessarily what the local population needed. The railway extended the industrialized Jeffrey Mine into the community, by carrying asbestos through the main streets of town night and day. Recognizing the dangers posed by the moving freight cars, JM officials sought, successfully, to close the main roads around the Jeffrey Mine for ten minutes several times each day.[5]

These local changes were connected to the growing global demand for the mineral (see Figure 8). By the end of the First World War, the province was providing 80 percent of the world's supply of asbestos.[6] In response to the high level of asbestos extraction in Quebec, the *Canadian Mining Journal* wrote that "the future of asbestos is only beginning, [and] the variety of its possible uses is immense, [so] that Canada, occupying such a dominating position in the asbestos market, may very well look forward

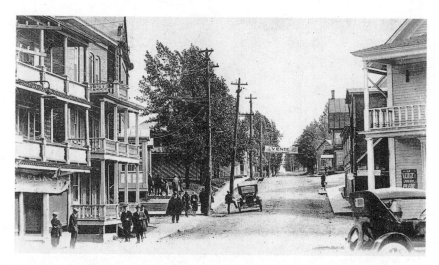

FIGURE 8   Sunday morning looking east along King Street, Asbestos, 1924
Source: WG Clark Fonds, ETRC

not only to a greater production of the raw material, but to multiplication
of the industries concerned with the manufacture and marketing of asbestos
in finished form."[7]

The town of Asbestos prospered following the war as demand for both
asbestos and asbestic skyrocketed. European postwar reconstruction counted
for a percentage of this escalation, but it was the American automobile
industry, which required asbestos for brake linings, that truly underpinned
the growth of the Jeffrey Mine. Growth was also stimulated by the increased
use of electricity, because asbestos was initially its most valuable insulator,[8]
and by new laws in some American states that banned wooden shingles
as a fire risk in the electrical age. As the *Canadian Mining Journal* noted
in 1920, the rise in demand for asbestic directly benefited operations at
the Jeffrey Mine, which was able to provide seemingly limitless amounts
of both long and short fibre.[9] In response to this market boom, JM announced that it was constructing a new manufacturing plant in Asbestos
that would require at least one hundred new employees.

American and British manufacturing plants imported approximately
$12,000,000 worth of raw asbestos in 1920, mainly from mines in Canada
and the southern half of Africa.[10] The new combination of resource extraction and product manufacturing in Asbestos followed the path that economic historian Harold Innis described in his staples thesis: small resource
communities in the Canadian hinterland remained exploited, economically

stunted places until they shifted from a foundation of simple resource extraction to one that included manufacturing. This shift began slowly in Asbestos in 1923, when JM opened the new manufacturing plant at the Jeffrey Mine, which consisted of two buildings, each 150 by 1,000 feet.[11] The plant was built at the beginning of what Quebec mining historian Marc Vallières calls the province's "technological revolution," which lasted until 1950 and offered job opportunities for more townspeople, including women.[12]

JM had transformed the pit into something resembling a machine "laid out in wide benches, [with] the rock being loaded into cars of standard gauge by steam-shovels and hauled on trains to the mill by steam locomotives on a maximum grade of three percent."[13] Jeffrey Mine workers now used the most technologically advanced steam-powered drills and shovels available. Benches were an especially efficient way to access ore in opencast mines; they were used in a variety of mineral and hardrock operations because this allowed for extraction on many different levels at once, besides preventing landslides when the edges of a pit became too steep. The company also pioneered the use of machinery in the pit: men who had once loaded chunks of broken rock into carting boxes at the bottom of the mine now operated steam shovels and other heavy equipment instead.[14]

The Jeffrey Mine was not the only modernizing aspect of Asbestos following the war. By 1922, the roads in Asbestos were congested due to the local population's increased reliance on automobiles, and the bridge leading to Danville was constantly being blocked by shipments from the mine. The situation worsened as fibre output increased. JM attempted to solve the problem by extending a road across company property as a transport route for trucks. JM soon after decided it needed to relocate the community's main road. Council approved JM's proposal to move part of the Asbestos-Danville road, having decided that the road was too close to the mine operations to be safe and that it was becoming an impediment to industrial progress, which was "so essential to the life and interest of the local community."[15] A new road was built by the company sixty-six feet from the edge of JM property.

Moving the road was a marker of prosperity, but it was also a great disruption to the townspeople, many of whom had to move their homes or businesses. Despite the disruption, only eight people in Asbestos – all of them local businessmen not directly affiliated with the mine – protested the move.[16] But the Jeffrey Mine was of vital importance to most of the community. All other possible land uses were secondary.

GROUNDBREAKING SUCCESS, 1924–38

The asbestos industry suffered from postwar overproduction in the early 1920s as global production increased. Declining prices forced many Quebec mines to shut down. JM temporarily closed the Jeffrey Mine in January 1924 because of overproduction, but the *Canadian Mining Journal* still reported that

> one can gain an idea of the magnitude of the mining operations of this company when one learns that eight big steam shovels are used in the amphitheatre-like open-cast workings; that to cope with the mine output, a new crushing plant had to be built, which will take care of 500 tons of rock per hour; and that a new mill ... is now ready to receive the crushed rock.[17]

The month-long closing of the mine froze the people of Asbestos, who were so dependent on the industry to support themselves and their families. The company made it clear that the closure would be short, and this promise sustained the local population through the month.

The Jeffrey Mine's closure was so short partly because of the booming automobile industry in the United States, which consumed more than 50 percent of all manufactured asbestos products for over a dozen uses.[18] JM, already a world leader in building materials, won contracts from the automobile, railway, and oil industries. The Jeffrey Mine was the company's largest and most profitable asbestos operation by far, and JM steadily increased its investment and presence in the town of Asbestos.

Anticipating further growth in the late 1920s due to the automobile industry's demand for the mineral, town council wrote to the Quebec government requesting permission to extend the boundaries of Asbestos for the future prosperity of the community. The request was granted, and the town soon covered eight hundred acres. JM immediately appealed for fifty-five acres of already settled town land around the mine in return for agreeing to continue supplying Asbestos with electricity.[19] In its request, the company explained that it had major expansion plans for the Jeffrey Mine operations, including covering all of the town's roads with gravel and constructing four new roads, which would be lined with houses for employees with families, equipped with such modern conveniences as running water, electricity, and streetlights.[20]

JM was bringing significant changes to the infrastructure of Asbestos, as well as to its culture (see Figure 9). In 1926, the company successfully

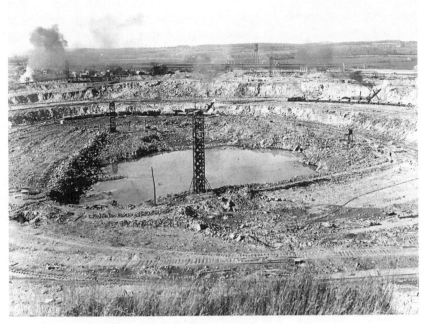

FIGURE 9   The Jeffrey Mine, 1928
Source: WG Clark Fonds, ETRC

lobbied the town council to introduce bilingual street signs in the community.[21] Asbestos was majority francophone, but the company officials
were anglophone and had an influence in local affairs that was larger than
their numbers. The linguistic divide in Asbestos closely followed the class
divide: the anglophone minority held power within the community because
of its managerial role at the Jeffrey Mine. Good relations between the
English and French in the community depended on good relations between
the managerial class and the working class at the mine. With record profits
for the industry, and with Asbestos's population growing to 3,602 by 1926,
local class relations were good, and the linguistic needs of JM and its officials were readily met by town council.

JM planned its fifty-five-acre expansion of the Jeffrey Mine operations
for 1928, but it was not completed until 1933 due to local resistance and
the changing global economy during the Great Depression. Now, for the
first time, the Jeffrey Mine began to significantly eat away at the town
beyond road closures and removals.[22] The enlargement of the pit destroyed
what locals referred to as the "nerve centre" of the community, including

Le Carré, the store opened in 1890 by the first mayor of Asbestos, Henri Roux.[23] JM gave the town an equal amount of land for the construction of a new commercial centre; even so, local merchants protested the expansion. JM's enlargement of the Jeffrey Mine changed not only the landscape but also the way townspeople related to it. A barbed wire fence around the pit now clearly separated land for work from land for living.

While many residents were upset about the destruction of the original section of the community, the late 1920s were exciting years in Asbestos and the expansion seemed a sign of greater things to come. In 1928, the region was internationally known as "the most important asbestos producing territory in the world. The asbestos mined there is the standard for the whole industry ... [and] with it all other asbestos is compared."[24] Land with this reputation could not be exploited enough, and the international reach of the Jeffrey Mine helped shape local dynamics.

All of this changed with the onset of the Great Depression, when the global price for asbestos declined sharply. JM controlled almost half of all the asbestos mined in Canada in the early 1930s. Now, with the onset of the economic crisis, it drastically reduced its workforce at the Jeffrey Mine, operating only one shift per day.[25] JM was strongly affected by the Depression because of its dependence on the collapsed automobile and construction industries. That the company combined mining and manufacturing in Asbestos did not help the situation: the community had been brought to a standstill, and local concerns about the mine's expansion into the town increased.

The town council defended the mine expansion by declaring that it would generate work for the community and sustain JM, which provided "almost all the revenue in Asbestos."[26] Even so, local physician Dr. Elzéar Émard made an official protest against the destruction of Le Carré in 1930, alleging that council was acting in the interests of JM, not the community.[27] Distance between the council and the company was necessary, especially in uncertain times. To quell accusations of partiality, the mayor appealed to the provincial government for a final decision on the expansion.

In 1931, the Quebec government, unwilling to obstruct any project that provided employment, sided with JM, and the first Bill of Expropriation for Asbestos was put into effect. Locals were forced to sell their land to the company. The community depended on the mine for its existence, and JM was in charge of that mine; it followed that the company was essentially in charge of Asbestos, and the expropriation solidified this. The local people's emotional attachment to community land, as evident in the protests over the expropriation, clearly did not matter. Under the rule of JM, the town did not have a history, as preserved in buildings or roads; rather, it had a future, which was to be achieved through unrestricted changes to the land. The expansion concluded in 1933.

The population of Asbestos had grown to 4,396 in 1931. Community affairs went on as normally as they could during the economic downturn. Town officials put their faith in the company and often asked JM officials for the use of company engineers when constructing new roads.[28] The property of many local merchants and homeowners had been severely damaged as the company moved roads and buildings to accommodate the growing Jeffrey Mine, and locals had to appeal directly to JM for compensation. Then the company closed operations at the mine and the mill between May 1932 and April 1933.

JM's efforts to develop new markets for magnesium pipe and boiler insulation yielded long-term success but could not compensate for the immediate decrease in demand for asbestos products within the auto industry.[29] The yearlong closure was hard on the people of Asbestos and forced many to rely on government assistance for survival. By the end of 1933, however the asbestos industry had bounced back, recording a 29 percent increase in production and a 71 percent increase in monetary value over the previous year.[30] Town council purchased additional acreage to prepare for community growth and to tap into a new water source now that the current one had become too contaminated. While production levels at the mine did not reach pre-Depression levels until after the Second World War, by 1935 employees were working an average of fifty-eight hours a week.

Canadian asbestos production continued to rise throughout the late 1930s. In 1936, it rose 43 percent in quantity and 41 percent in value over the previous year,[31] producing 247,954 metric tons worth $9,958,183. In 1937, Canada produced 337,443 metric tons of asbestos worth $14,505,541.[32] JM's manufacturing plants at Asbestos and Montreal could handle only 5 percent of the fibre being extracted from the Jeffrey Mine. The rest of the output went to the several hundred factories the company ran in the United States, the world's leading exporter of finished asbestos products.[33]

In the first issue of the bilingual *Johns-Manville News Pictorial*, which was distributed to local employees each month between 1938 and 1949, the company tried to assure workers of the industry's stability. It also highlighted the connection of people to land in Asbestos by focusing on the work of men like Achille Boudreau and Joe Letarte. Boudreau was photographed sitting in the pit wearing his denim jacket as he cobbed asbestos fibres out of large pieces of rock by breaking it along the fibrous seams with a hammer. Latarte, also a cobber, was pictured climbing out of the pit with a bucket of rock in one hand and a burlap bag full of hand-picked fibre slung over his shoulder as though he was an asbestos Santa.[34]

As the industry recovered from the Depression, many asbestos communities in the region found it difficult to meet the increased demand because there was no physical space on which to expand operations. This was not the case in Asbestos, where industry trumped community when it came to issues of land use. In 1938, JM appealed to town council with a proposal to expand the Jeffrey Mine once again, this time onto fourteen undeveloped lots. Council immediately approved the company's request.[35]

INDUSTRIAL REVOLUTION
MEETS NATURAL PHENOMENON, 1938–49

The years following the Depression taught the people of Asbestos that if they put their faith in the Jeffrey Mine and JM, they would prosper. The 1938 expansion did not directly affect the homes and businesses of the town and thus was not as controversial as the first major enlargement. It was clear to the local population that the pit had almost reached its physical limits, for it resembled a steep inverted cone with limited access to fibre at the bottom.[36] Due to the threat of landslides, workers could only dig deeper for so long without first expanding wider. For the structural stability of the land and the financial stability of the town, the Jeffrey Mine had to expand its girth.

Townspeople and the town council viewed the expansion as an example of progress after the economic trials of the early 1930s. To compensate for lost space, council purchased seven unused lots from local farmers in January 1939, then fourteen more the following spring.[37] The town needed more land to accommodate the growing workforce and to address the shrinking community space. Clearly, it was learning to balance the two interdependent aspects of Asbestos. The purchases were well-timed. In 1939, JM and town council significantly developed the land surrounding the community, and the *Canadian Mining Journal* declared the Jeffrey Mine the largest chrysotile asbestos mine in the world (see Figure 10).[38]

Local understandings of place and self in Asbestos were rooted in an industrialized landscape that was constantly in flux. The original hill on which Jeffrey and Webb found their first deposits of asbestos had almost

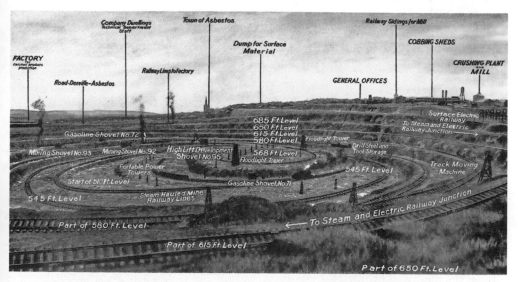

FIGURE 10   Mining and haulage arrangement of levels and approaches at the
Jeffrey Mine, 1939
Source: RC Rowe, "Mining and Milling Operations of the Canadian Johns-Manville
Company Ltd. at Asbestos, PQ," *The Canadian Mining Journal*, April 1939, 193

disappeared by 1939, but the bottom of the pit remained about 750 feet
above sea level and was 510 feet deep and 300 feet wide, with spiralling
benches thirty-five feet high and at least seventy-five feet wide to accommodate the trucks and trains emerging from the bottom.[39] According to
the *Canadian Mining Journal*, the land in Asbestos told a tale of large-scale
progress:

> The first impression gathered from a tour of these workings is one of size.
> Here is an operation that handles great quantities of material, and uses
> mammoth machines in the process. [Here] is the largest power shovel in
> Canada; along its levels run standard locomotives hauling trains of cars ...
> Yet as one stands on the high side of the pit looking down, these great
> machines look like toys in that immensity of space. It is a big job worked
> in a big way because some 3,000,000 tons of rock and stripping are handled
> from the pit in a year.[40]

The Jeffrey Mine was now a natural and a technological phenomenon.
Derricks mounted around the mine now held the drills that made blasting holes in five separate working areas of the pit to ensure precision and

to cut back on staff. When JM officials came up with this cost-saving idea, drill manufacturers told them that replacing men with machines was impossible,[41] so the company invented new machinery to do it. This further revolutionized the intersection of land and technology in the Jeffrey Mine.

Locomotives now carried steel, drill bits, explosives, and other supplies around the pit. Three four-yard electric shovels worked in tandem with one eight-yard shovel to load the fibre into empty train cars heading to the surface.

For all that, people still laboured in the pit. Groups of men operated machines and packed explosives into the mechanically drilled holes before taking cover. Employees also moved the pumps that extracted the estimated 500,000 gallons of surface and underground water that filled the pit each day, and picked through the rubble after blasting to remove any pieces of wood, blasting wire, or other foreign objects that would decrease the value of the mineral packaged at the mill. Shifts operated twenty-four hours a day; workers appeared ant-like under the 1,000-watt floodlights that shone on the Jeffrey Mine at night.

The connection between the people of Asbestos and the mine was changing with the increased industrialization of the land, but it was not disappearing. Both Richard White and Thomas G. Andrews have written detailed histories on the connections workers forge with the natural environment they alter and shape each day, and Asbestos is yet another example of this pattern.[42] Jeffrey Mine workers were permanently changing the land with their hands and with machines, but in doing so, they were not distancing themselves from the natural rhythms of the environment. Instead, they were developing a deep and unique understanding of the mineral and the rock that surrounded it. The sounds, smells, and dust emerging from the mine twenty-four hours a day were a steady presence in Asbestos. They were a constant reminder that this small town was part of a global industry – one described by the 1939 American *Minerals Yearbook* as indispensible to modern life – on which it depended, but that also depended on it.[43]

The outbreak of the Second World War marked the beginning of a thirty-year boom for both the mineral and the community. By 1941, JM sales had increased by 50 percent because of wartime industries and the temporary disappearance of Soviet fibre from competition.[44] The closing of European markets during the war did not severely affect the company or its operations at Asbestos because its foundations were in Canada and the United States, both of which continued to feed the machines of war with the fireproof mineral. The American wartime industrial boom more than compensated for the loss of European sales, and workers at the Jeffrey Mine often had trouble keeping up with demand.

These were exciting times for Asbestos. JM and other manufacturing companies were constantly developing new technologies and products that contained Jeffrey Mine fibre. This included asbestos cement, which saw asbestic added to cement to reinforce its strength and durability and led many contemporaries to believe that the "Asbestos Age" was just beginning.[45] Asbestos cement was especially popular in the American construction industry, and the Jeffrey Mine's short asbestic fibre was ideal for this product.

At the end of 1941, JM approached town council to purchase part of two roads for mine expansion. Although this area bordered a central area of the community, council granted the request in the spring of 1942 – at this time of great local prosperity, the company could do no wrong.[46] JM gave the town $5,000 for sacrificing less than five hundred feet of road. The lack of protest from local residents suggests that most of the community agreed that mine expansion was a positive thing. However, local homeowner Joseph A. Lambert immediately asked council for permission to move his house away from the planned expansion at his own expense. Not everyone was thrilled to be living in such close proximity to the noise and dust that was produced by the Jeffrey Mine twenty-four hours a day. Between June 1942 and February 1943, four other residents made similar requests.[47] These moves indicate that the community managed the land with a quiet acceptance. Rather than try to prevent mine expansion or sue the company for the costs associated with relocation, the residents simply moved out of the way.

Whenever the Jeffrey Mine "ate" part of the town, there was a rollback effect – the town moved homes and purchased new land on the edges of the community. Most JM officials lived on a knoll far from the Jeffrey Mine and owned cars that took them from their homes to the pit each day. Workers, on the other hand, usually walked to the mine, and many rented affordable housing from JM close to the edges of the pit. The families in these homes were moved at JM's expense when the company expanded the mine; local homeowners placed their houses on logs and relocated them by horse when the mine grew. In June 1942, town council annexed a large portion of unused farmland in order to expand the livable limits of Asbestos.

The expansion provided new land for those displaced by the growing mine, as well as space for new residents who had moved to the community to work for JM. The mine was an excellent source of wartime employment. Three shifts kept operations going twenty-four hours a day, seven days a week, and still the mine could not meet the market demand. The wartime reduction in male employees allowed more women into JM operations, until by 1943, 25 percent of the workers at the manufacturing plant were female.[48] This offered a new way of life to a significant portion of the population.

By 1943, the Jeffrey Mine encompassed 115 acres of land, and local workers were extracting 6,000 tons of rock and mineral daily. Despite these impressive figures, JM was unable to expand the mine quickly enough to meet industrial demand when the United States went to war in 1941. The mine had grown so close to the residential portion of Asbestos that sewage began pouring into the pit, contaminating the fibre.[49] JM had to develop a new way of looking at the land. The US *Minerals Yearbook* stated that the global shortage of asbestos fibre was the result of the opencast mines like the one at Asbestos.[50] Although opencast operations were the preferred method of extraction for asbestos mining companies, the presence of townspeople surrounding these pits often slowed growth, resulting in time-consuming negotiations every few years. Recognizing that the demand and the price for asbestos were both high enough to defray the costs of changing how workers extracted the mineral from the Jeffrey Mine, the president of C-JM, G.K. Foster decided to take operations underground.

Underground mining allowed JM to expand its operations and increase production quickly without infringing on the townspeople's property, because shafts took up far less land than an open pit. Underground operations also hid the drastic changes to the land that opencast mining put on display. The first two shafts at the Jeffrey Mine were ten by ten feet and about 750 feet deep, and each had a conveyor belt twenty-five feet high leading out of the ground towards the mills.[51] No longer would asbestos-containing rocks be blasted out of the pit into the town: instead, they would slowly be carried up to the surface after being broken free underground.

Town council approved the building of these shafts; in return, JM donated company land to extend one of the community's main roads. JM also built the Hotel Iroquois beside the shafts to house two hundred single male workers who had been hired to meet the rising global demand for asbestos fibre. Canadian asbestos production rose by more than 100,000 short tons during the Second World War, and there was little fear among industry insiders that the market would collapse after the war because the mineral was so much in demand for peacetime uses.[52] In its transition from wartime to peacetime markets, JM invested more money in Asbestos to expand production.

The company's development of shaft mining, combined with mill expansion, increased JM's profits by 50 percent in the postwar period.[53] Underground mining required less space, increased overall yields, and ensured the highest quality of asbestos taken from the mine by protecting it from the elements. Combined with opencast methods, underground operations allowed JM to increase production without expanding the pit farther into the community. This improved company-community relations; but one group that JM could not appease, however, was local merchants.

There was constant tension between the company and the smaller businessmen of Asbestos. Following the destruction of Le Carré and its neighbouring businesses in the first major expansion of 1928–33, local merchants attempted to create a new centre on rue Bourbeau. It was here and on a neighbouring road that JM chose to build its first mining shafts. In return, JM offered to extend another road for the merchants and to provide any help it could to "defend the interests of the City of Asbestos." But business owners along rue Bourbeau were not satisfied.[54] La Ligue des Propriétaires d'Asbestos Inc. presented a statement to council entreating them to block any JM operation that threatened rue Bourbeau (and therefore the value of their properties and businesses), using every legal measure available.[55] This was real conflict over land use in Asbestos, and it suggests the difficulties of maintaining harmonious community relations in single-resource and single-company towns. Local businessmen were primarily concerned with the loss of property values and revenues, but JM's land management provided the community with stability and profits. Council ended the meeting without making a decision, thus postponing having to choose between the company and local businessmen.

JM promised compensation for any damages attributable to the closing of rue Bourbeau, but local merchants continued to protest the change in land use. They believed that townspeople would not shop next to mining shafts and conveyor belts connected to the noisy mill. They were concerned for their properties, but their commercial future as independent businessmen was even more important to them. By January 1947, Mayor Albert Goudreau had had enough of the debate, demanding that council make a firm decision on the subject with the community's economic future in mind. Council approved JM's request to close the road.[56]

Town council recognized the importance of accommodating JM's industrial and environmental needs, especially given that the Canadian asbestos industry was booming due to European postwar reconstruction.[57]

Anticipating that more people would be moving to Asbestos to work at the Jeffrey Mine, council also moved to acquire new land on which to grow. Between September 1947 and January 1949, the town purchased land from the county, local property owners, and even JM, which held several lots that did not contain profitable amounts of asbestos.[58] The town was growing in the postwar period, and so was the industry.

In 1947, the Quebec industry exported 10,785,189 tons of fibre valued at $438,356,805.[59] With the combination of open pit mining, shaft mining, and a new block-caving system the company had introduced, extraction levels at the Jeffrey Mine far surpassed those of its regional competitors. Block-caving is a form of underground mining particularly suited to land that already has a steep, working opencast pit. Jeffrey Mine workers undercut the benches that spiralled up the Jeffrey Mine and drilled and blasted into the rock above. Workers operated giant double-drum mechanical slushers that scraped the rock out of these caves and brought it to the surface, loading the ore onto train cars to be taken to the factory. The space inside each "block" was limited to between ten by twenty feet and ten by thirty-five feet. Cave-ins were a constant threat, and each block was two hundred feet from the one beside it in an attempt to prevent them from collapsing. Block-caving further industrialized the land without visible signs from above. It also changed the structure of the Jeffrey Mine, weakening the benches on which trains and trucks brought men and mineral to the surface.

By 1948, the dimensions of the opencast pit had grown substantially, to 3,200 feet long by 2,800 feet wide, reaching the absolute limits of JM property. Underground mining allowed the company to continue operations without purchasing more land from the town or risking landslides. It also enabled workers to extract between 19,000 and 22,760 tons of rock every twenty-four hours.[60] As a reminder, just ten years earlier, when only opencast methods were used, workers at the Jeffrey Mine had extracted only 389,688 tons per annum.[61] The Jeffrey Mine was now run on electricity and coal-fuelled steam power, which significantly boosted extraction levels.

The Jeffrey Mine had become increasingly industrialized over the first half of the twentieth century, and marks of this industrialization were visible throughout Asbestos. Railway lines, new roads, new neighbourhoods, workers being replaced by machines that caused more noise and dust to come from the pit, and town council's willingness to rule in favour of JM when it came to local land use issues, were all signs of the widespread industrialization of the land and community. To remain competitive in the global asbestos industry, the local population had to sacrifice town infrastructure and space to accommodate the mine's need for more mineral-rich land.

While town council focused on the success of the local industry, competing ideologies slowly developed over how community land should be used. The labour of Jeffrey Mine workers had helped JM succeed. It had also connected townspeople to the land, and many believed they had a right to decide how their property and community space should be used. In January 1949, council purchased 55,125 square feet of land to accommodate the growing population.[62] These plans were put on hold when Jeffrey Mine workers went on strike to ensure that their voice in the community – and the international industry it fed – was maintained despite the rapid industrialization of the pit. The labour dispute, which folded together issues of land use, human health, and community, would radically change the way the natural environment was used and understood in Asbestos.

3

Negotiating Risk, 1918–49

I N 1995, DR. GERRIT W.H. Schepers published an article on the time he had spent at the Saranac Laboratory in Saranac Lake, New York. Interning there as a postdoctoral student in 1949, Schepers discovered the autopsied lungs of at least nine "Quebec Asbestos Workers" that Quebec Asbestos Mining Association (QAMA) attorney Yvan Sabourin had smuggled to the lab from Asbestos and Thetford between 1944 and 1946. QAMA had deemed a study of these lungs necessary because "workers had begun to agitate for compensation [for their asbestos-related diseases, and] ... such a large number of cases in such a small and well-defined group of industrial employees suggested a significant problem."[1] The lungs Sabourin delivered had come from deceased retirees. These retirees had been secretly autopsied; their lungs had been illegally brought across an international border, dissected, placed on nameless slides, studied, and filed away. It is unclear whether the researchers at Saranac Lake knew the circumstances by which these lungs had been obtained, but they were eager to discover what they could reveal about asbestos-related disease. As the primary funding body for asbestos studies at Saranac, JM oversaw any publications emerging from the lab on asbestos, and prevented Schepers from publishing on his discovery for decades.

Although the people of Asbestos did not know of these autopsies or of the specific diseases researchers were finding in the bodies of their deceased coworkers, family members, and friends, they were constantly negotiating the health risks of living next to the world's largest chrysotile asbestos mine. Some risks, such as those to the miners themselves, were considered acceptable. Others, like those to the women and children of the community, were not. The diseases caused by asbestos are painful and debilitating. Those affected would have known they were sick, but they remained unaware of the types of illnesses asbestos caused and could not make a direct, certain link between their symptoms and their occupations. Company officials may have defended themselves by saying they did not want to unnecessarily alarm the workforce with premature publicity about the research project at Saranac Lake; even so, it remains significant that the townspeople had no idea that JM was using the community as a giant research laboratory, with workers and their families acting as test mice.

The Jeffrey Mine was the economic, geographic, and cultural heart of Asbestos, bringing it both life and death. The community celebrated and suffered through the extremes of the asbestos industry, from its meteoric rise as "one of Nature's most marvellous productions"[2] to its startling collapse brought about by the health risks associated with it. This history can be roughly defined by periods of public ignorance and public outrage. It is also marked by an unwavering local commitment to the success of the Jeffrey Mine.

This chapter examines the medical histories of the people of Asbestos between 1918 and 1949, the year in which workers were part of an exposé about the scientific evidence of risks associated with asbestos, risks that had become a major international issue. From 1929 onwards, JM suppressed medical studies on the dangers of the mineral, employees coughed up dust after only short periods of work, and generations slowly suffocated to death because of the long-term bodily effects the industry had on the community. In much the same way that the tobacco industry later sought to suppress and contradict evidence of the harm caused by cigarettes, JM denied and fudged the medical evidence of asbestos's baneful effects on human bodies. This was a period in which townspeople were inclined to trust in medical professionals, company officials, and the land over local bodily knowledge.

DISCOVERY AND DENIAL, 1918 TO 1930

Soon after JM purchased the Jeffrey Mine, it brought its own medical professionals to the community and established a local clinic for employees. These doctors were anglophone, and furthermore, they often reported the health conditions of Jeffrey Mine workers to company officials in New York rather than to the patients themselves.[3] Company doctors often contributed to a paternalistic control over most aspects of local life.[4] There were a few independent doctors in Asbestos, but the lives of JM employees were oriented towards the Jeffrey Mine, and they had free yearly check-ups at the company clinic. Few local residents felt the need to seek an independent medical opinion. JM had a vested interest in the bodies of the people of Asbestos, and their doctors were fundamental to the preservation of a calm, if not exactly healthy, workforce.

JM also had doctors stationed in its processing towns, such as Manville, New Jersey, but Jeffrey Mine workers were a major concern because the mine was JM's main source of asbestos. Nowhere else were JM employees exposed to such a pure, raw form of the mineral, and company doctors could monitor the progression of disease in Asbestos in order to see the effects of the mineral on human health, untainted by other materials. The JM clinic also ensured that the health issues of JM employees in Asbestos would be addressed differently than elsewhere in the province, free from the administrative hand that the Catholic Church, and later, the provincial government, traditionally wielded in medical care. Asbestos was a single-industry and single-company town, and employees trusted JM with their health the same way they trusted the company with the mine.

In 1924, JM opened Canada's first mineral processing factory in Asbestos. This increased profits, provided employment opportunities for women and children, and created more mineral dust than the community had ever experienced. That same year, Dr. W.E. Cooke reported in the *British Medical Journal* that Nellie Kershaw, who processed the fibre for Turner Brothers Asbestos in Rochdale, England, had died because of her exposure to the mineral. Cooke explained that asbestos caused a fatal hardening of the lungs,[5] but the Quebec community was unaware of this discovery, or of the dangers the dusty new factory would bring. In 1927, Cooke coined the term "asbestosis" to describe the hardening effect the mineral had on human lungs.[6] A year earlier, JM had received its first claim for compensation from textile factory workers in New Jersey suffering from what Cooke would call asbestosis.[7]

In Quebec, an increased public focus on tuberculosis (the incidence of which had risen significantly during the war years) inspired an aggressive health education program on respiratory disease. Also, Louis-Alexandre Taschereau's provincial government acted on the recommendations of the Royal Commission on Labour and made it mandatory for companies to carry insurance against compensation claims.[8] Following this regulation, JM purchased the necessary insurance from the Sun Life Assurance Co.

In 1926, Sun Life medical director Dr. G.W. Wright wrote that both companies could protect themselves by funding the establishment of a Department of Industrial Hygiene at McGill University in Montreal. Sun Life and JM, wrote Wright, could provide "guidance in regard to matters affecting community or individual health – such as, aid in preparation of publicity, occasional research matters ... field investigations ... or industrial hazards ... The usefulness of the University could be made apparent in relation to group insurance much more readily than in any other way."[9] McGill established the department with this funding, and the university forged a long-standing – but unofficial – working relationship with JM.

In 1929, Metropolitan Life Assurance, which had taken over JM's insurance policy from Sun Life, urged Frank G. Pedley, one of the only doctors in Canada publishing on asbestos-related disease, to approach McGill and "enter into an agreement ... to secure for the Company certain services and information relating to the health of industrial workers."[10] Pedley wrote of his new relationship with JM that "such a plan involves a definite quid pro quo, payments specifically conditioned upon a commensurate return,"[11] and as the top expert on asbestos-related disease in Canada at the time, he was an important researcher to lead the study.

At the beginning of the Great Depression, the death rate in Quebec was higher for francophones than for anglophones. This was partly because of poor medical care among relatively impoverished French Canadians, but it also had something to do with their greater engagement in industrial activity. This was a population that worked hard and suffered for it, but because of JM, the situation at Asbestos seemed different, with leading medical professionals visiting the community to monitor workers' health.

With the founding of McGill's new Department of Industrial Hygiene, in 1930 Pedley was invited by the university and JM to work with company doctor R.H. Stevenson to assess the health status of Jeffrey Mine employees. In his short report published in the *Canadian Medical Journal*, Pedley summarized his findings:

> asbestos is a mineral of interest to Canadian physicians ... If work with asbestos presented a hazard to the worker it would be reasonable to suppose that cases of disease would be reported from time to time, but so far as can be determined no cases of specific disease have been reported among asbestos workers in the Province of Quebec.[12]

This was what Pedley published. That published report had been thoroughly edited by JM and Metropolitan Life officials and completely misrepresented his findings, which Pedley found frustrating.[13] His study of workers at both Asbestos and Thetford had revealed a very different story. Pedley's lengthy, detailed, unpublished report offers a very different first look at how the industry was affecting the bodies of the people of Asbestos and at how medical reports on the mineral's effects on human health were tightly controlled by the industry.

Pedley's study was flawed from the beginning. He misleadingly compared Jeffrey Mine workers to those at Thetford's asbestos mines. Every JM employee had to pass a physical exam before he or she began working at the Jeffrey Mine. Thetford did not have this restriction.[14] Subsequently diagnosed medical problems among JM employees could therefore be counted as having occurred during their time at the mine, which was important for compensation claims and for injuries such as hernias, from which four men at Asbestos suffered in 1930. Furthermore, while Pedley studied 141 men at Asbestos and only 54 at Thetford, the majority of those at the Jeffrey Mine had worked in the industry for fewer than nine years. Members of the Thetford sample averaged more than fifteen years of mine work. Furthermore, most Jeffrey Mine workers were between fifteen and forty years of age, while most of those at Thetford were over forty, and there was no dusty factory there. Because asbestos-related diseases typically took at least ten years of heavy industrial exposure to present to doctors in the 1930s, these were crucial differences.[15]

Pedley acknowledged that the design of his research would likely show higher rates of disability and disease in Thetford, but he made no effort to compensate for the disparity. He found no occurrences of what British investigators called "asbestos corns" on Jeffrey Mine employees, but admitted that he was uncertain of what these small, "pin head sized elevations of the skin, somewhat like minute warts," caused by fibrous slivers, actually looked like.[16] Twenty-seven men in Asbestos had infected tonsils, but Pedley failed to connect this to the dusty conditions in which they worked. Pedley may have been the Canadian authority on asbestos-related disease, but this was a small field, and compared to his counterparts in Britain and the United States, Pedley was far from expert.

This became increasingly apparent when Pedley focused on the lungs of the men at Asbestos. When examining the 101 prescreened X-rays that JM's doctor in Asbestos gave him, Pedley found only four cases of "definite" asbestosis, but immediately discounted these because "none of the cases of asbestosis appeared to suffer from disabling symptoms. Perhaps the most common symptom was shortness of breath," but according to the clinic notes given to him by JM's doctor, "less than half the cases complained of this" and "very few of the men were coughing."[17] The workers were not complaining of disease, so seemingly there was no cause for alarm. Pedley augmented X-rays that were difficult to read with a test to measure chest expansion, using nothing but a tape measure and a sheet covering the employee's torso, but he soon gave this up because of its inaccuracy.

According to Pedley, "conversation with physicians and mine managers in the asbestos regions indicated that no hazard to health was suspected in connection with work in the asbestos mining and milling industry."[18] He also noted that "it is the general impression both among miners and physicians that asbestos dust is not particularly harmful ... From the public health standpoint ... it seems hardly likely that asbestosis will become of importance either from the standpoint of morbidity or mortality."[19] The leading medical professional publishing on asbestos in the country, Pedley depended heavily on conclusions reached by company doctors. He also believed that asbestosis was not the terribly painful affliction reported by British workers, and he seemed convinced that because it was confined to the working class, it did not present a risk to the general public. All of this had profound effects on how the people of Asbestos, company doctors, and JM understood health. Disease is both biologically and socially constructed, and neither Pedley nor anyone associated with Asbestos was ready to conclude that asbestos-related disease was a concern.

"THE LESS SAID ABOUT ASBESTOS, THE BETTER OFF WE ARE": 1930–40

Still, JM was worried. Although few men at the Jeffrey Mine had severe cases of asbestosis in 1930, the fact that almost half of those studied in Thetford did[20] suggested that it was only a matter of time before the same occurred in Asbestos. The mineral had gained a global reputation that was synonymous with safety, and manufacturers were constantly adding it to new products such as oxygen bottles in airplanes and hospital ceiling tiles.[21] JM would not sacrifice its profits for the sake of its workers. Instead, company officials believed they could control the problem. In a 1931 letter between JM vice-presidents, E.M. Voorhees wrote S.A. Williams that "ever since dust suits have been brought against us at Manville [New Jersey] we have considered, first, the possibility of installing the most modern and improved dust collecting systems."[22] Although this technology was expensive, it promised to be less costly than the occupational health and safety lawsuits that JM's American employees were beginning to launch against the company.

In a 1931 letter from Metropolitan Life to JM attorneys, a Dr. McConnell wrote that Pedley's unpublished report, "like the report on the American plants, will be given no publicity by us except with the consent of the firms concerned."[23] Both Met Life and JM were aware of the potential cost of compensation claims were Pedley's full report to be released. This awareness led the company to go on the offensive: the medical knowledge its doctors discovered would be kept secret, and the evidence of others would be denied. There were few independent doctors in Asbestos, and JM employees had mandatory, free yearly checkups at the company clinic. So it was extremely rare for a doctor outside of JM control to examine Jeffrey Mine employees, and as a consequence, it seems probable that asbestos-related diseases went underreported and unacknowledged by both the company and the workers for years.

After Pedley submitted his report to JM,[24] the company began a campaign against those who claimed that asbestos was detrimental to human health. Because the asbestos-related deaths of British factory workers could not be ignored, JM claimed that it was African crocidolite asbestos that was dangerous, not Canadian chrysotile,[25] and insisted that Jeffrey Mine asbestos was completely safe. British doctors immediately refuted this claim, stating that 80 percent of the asbestos used in England came from Canada.[26] Yet JM would maintain the argument for decades. So forceful was the company's insistence that Canadian asbestos was harmless that it permeated the local community and convinced townspeople that the mineral and their land were safe.

While publicly denying that asbestos caused severe health effects, the company was in an internal panic over the potential lawsuits that its employees could launch against it. Company officials knew that the key to a healthy workforce at the Jeffrey Mine – and therefore proof that the Canadian mineral was safe – was the efficient removal of dust from the factory air. Some steps were taken. In a letter to S.A. Williams, Jeffrey Mine vice-president C.H. Shoemaker wrote that "since September 1931, no new dust collection equipment has been installed in the factory, chiefly because the equipment there meets 'all practical requirements' [and] inspection by the medical officers of the Quebec Board of Health 'indicates a clear ticket.'"[27] According to Shoemaker, existing measures, including respirators and extractor fans, eliminated 80 percent of the dust in the factory and mill, but this estimate reflected optimum circumstances. Some workers refused to wear breathing apparatus, saying that "[they] do not find respirators practicable." Reflecting on this, Shoemaker opined that "the dust in the mills is evidently less irritating and is more fibrous than in [other] locations, resulting in less need for a respirator and more trouble with the filter clogging when a respirator is used."[28]

Shoemaker's sentiments reflected those of Pedley two years earlier: the workers did not complain, so there was no cause for concern. Respirator technology was constantly improving, and JM urged employees to use the devices, but it did not mandate their use at the Jeffrey Mine until 1975. Clogged filters remained a problem, but many workers elected not to wear respirators, or they did not demand better dust control measures. The lack of action by Jeffrey Mine workers reveals an acceptance of dust, as they understood it at the time, in Asbestos. As historian Geoffrey Tweedale explains in his work on the British asbestos industry, "dust was an accepted fact of life in many industries, besides asbestos," and because they were not informed of the very real dangers concerning it, workers had no reason to fear it any more than they feared other types of dust.[29]

Although Jeffrey Mine workers did not know what asbestos dust was doing to their bodies, an increasing number of medical professionals did. Members of the British medical community wrote much of the literature emerging on asbestos-related disease because the deaths of British factory workers had convinced them that the mineral was not safe. In 1933, the Chief Inspector of Factories in Britain, Dr. E.R.A. Merewether, stated that "if only the slightest exposure to the dust results ultimately in death, then the scope of the necessary preventive measures is summed up in one word – prohibition – for, practically speaking, it is impossible to prevent such exposure."[30] But rather than pushing for prohibition, Mereweather encouraged a strict regime of dust control to reduce risk. If dust could not be sufficiently controlled by ventilation machines, he encouraged the use of respirators as a second line of defence. The mineral was too important to the industrial and economic development of the Western world, especially during the Great Depression, to prohibit its trade. Supporting Merewether's view of the mineral, Frank Pedley, who was still at McGill, but who had distanced himself from JM, published a report in the *Canadian Medical Association Journal* in 1933 that stated that asbestosis worked twice as fast as, and with symptoms more severe than, silicosis, a similar industrial disease.[31]

To contradict these damning reports, JM funded medical professionals to lead studies demonstrating that asbestos was safe. Writing to Metropolitan Life's assistant medical director, Dr. A.J. Lanza, in 1933, the director of Saranac Laboratory, Dr. Leroy Gardner, stated that "the fat seems to be in the fire" because of leaked medical reports on JM factory workers in New Jersey that resulted in compensation claims.[32] If successful, these claims had the potential to result in others and in a growing awareness of the dangers of asbestos. New health and safety measures were put in place at the factory in Manville, New Jersey, and JM vice-president Vandiver Brown wrote to his brother, president Lewis H. Brown, that during the rest of 1933, they must "bring other operations, especially Waukegan, Alexandria, Lompoc, and Asbestos to Manville efficiency."[33] Dust control at the Jeffrey Mine was in serious need of improvement, but the people of Asbestos were more secluded than those who worked at JM's American plants because of language barriers and a lack of concern for industrial disease within the Canadian medical community. This seclusion allowed the company a degree of freedom – and delay – when it came to dust control measures.

While factories were slowly brought up to health standards, company-funded doctors worked to dispel the idea that asbestos was a dangerous mineral. In an address to the Home Office Life Underwriters Association in November 1933, Lanza claimed, "I am going to make this a little bit dramatic. So far as we could ascertain, there is no dust hazard or asbestos hazard in connection with the actual mining or quarrying operations … In the open pit and quarry work there was no apparent pulmonary hazard."[34] Lanza continued to spread this claim in high-profile medical journals in the years that followed.[35] In 1934, Lanza met with Metropolitan Life officials to discuss the elimination of dust in factories. During the meeting, he insisted that knowledge of asbestos-related disease was still too rudimentary to prove that the mineral posed a serious health risk.[36]

The corporate suppression of knowledge relating to the dangers asbestos posed to human health continued for several decades. In the 1930s, JM diminished the severity of asbestosis in industry-funded – and edited – medical reports, which the company also used as evidence against compensation claims initiated in the United States. The company feigned injury from "the shyster lawyer[s] and the quack doctor[s]"[37] who were launching lawsuits against them. The president of Raybestos-Manhattan, Sumner Simpson, cautioned JM officials against this tactic and warned that "the less said about asbestos, the better off we are."[38]

Simpson urged caution because in the mid-1930s, unions in both America and Quebec, including the Fédération nationale des employés de l'industrie minière, were becoming more knowledgeable about asbestos-related disease. As a result, JM asked Saranac's Dr. Leroy Gardner to study the effects of asbestos dust on mice. Gardner was paid for the study on the condition that JM had the right to "determine whether, to what extent and in what manner [his conclusions] shall be made public."[39] Officials of other asbestos-producing companies in JM's network, aware of how dangerous the mineral actually was, were worried about the possible negative outcomes of Gardner's study. Simpson made this concern clear when he wrote that "the reports may be so favorable to us that they would cause us no trouble, but they might be just the opposite; which could be very embarrassing."[40] Industry leaders did not want – or need – yet another study to further prove the dangers of asbestos.

Gardner agreed to the conditions the company set for his study. Meanwhile, JM's doctor in Asbestos became another spokesman for the industry. Dr. R.H. Stevenson had helped Pedley in his 1930 examination of Jeffrey Mine employees, but it was not until 1938 – after Quebec officially recognized asbestosis as an industrial disease due to pressure from the Fédération nationale des employés de l'industrie minière,[41] – that JM asked him to take a more public role. In his May 23, 1938, address to Quebec's asbestos producers, Stevenson defended the health record of the Canadian industry and insisted that it was only African crocidolite asbestos that caused disease because of its high silica content (silica was absent in Jeffrey Mine chrysotile). Stevenson stated that asbestosis was "a rare case among asbestos workers" in North America and that this "has been experimentally proved by ... Dr. L.U. Gardner of [the] Trudeau Laboratory at Saranac. There is very little clinical evidence of Asbestosis [sic], and certainly not enough to even venture a diagnosis."[42] Gardner's research on the effects of asbestos dust on rodents was being used by JM to defend the mineral in Quebec even before he had finished his study.

Stevenson also relied on his own experience in Asbestos to show that the mineral was safe. He said he had been studying asbestosis there for ten years, and "we have been highly pleased to note the extreme rarity of asbestosis among our men ... As is to be expected the cases discovered showing early Asbestosis [sic] were men who had worked a long time in the company service."[43] For Stevenson, asbestosis was not a deadly respiratory disease, but rather a part of getting old in the industry, like wrinkles or a bad back. Those who suffered from it at the Jeffrey Mine were mostly men who worked in the mill, which convinced Stevenson "that it is a good idea to transfer men away from the mill after ten to twelve years of service to other departments. You will see ... that our position is very far from serious as far as actual damage to the men is concerned."[44]

Rotating mill workers every ten years or so did not prevent the progression of asbestos-related disease in Jeffrey Mine workers. Asbestosis begins with shortness of breath and leads to a slow and painful death due to suffocation. For Stevenson to say the condition of the men with asbestosis at the Jeffrey Mine was not serious was misleading, and his direct inter-action with workers influenced the way they understood what was hap-pening to their bodies. According to Stevenson, the good health of Asbestos men, at least during their first decade on the job, proved that the mineral, and the industry, was safe.

Despite Stevenson's claims, many of Quebec's asbestos producers still had doubts. C.S. Bell, lawyer for British asbestos manufacturing company Turner and Newall, which owned a mine in Thetford, but also interests in African mines, forwarded a transcript of the speech to his employers. A note from Bell included with the speech stated that while Stevenson "appears to consider that Rhodesian asbestos is more liable to promote Asbestosis [sic] than Canadian, by reason of the higher proportion of SiO_2 ... as far as I can trace from the published analyses the Silica content of Canadian and Rhodesian fibre is almost identical, i.e. about 40%."[45] Experience dealing with health problems in British factories trumped Stevenson's convictions, but Turner and Newall officials did not publicly refute his claims. The unwillingness of company officials to challenge Stevenson's assertion that Canadian asbestos was safe quickly became a much-relied on mantra in defence of Quebec's mines.

Still JM worried about growing health issues in Asbestos. In 1938, the company's board of directors reported internally that the dust collection equipment at the Jeffrey Mine's mill was only 50 percent effective. Mineral dust hovered like clouds over the community, being in general an "almost intolerable nuisance," with complaints rising from both the town council and individuals.[46] JM officials reported that "so heavy at times was the concentration of this dust in the mill area that it began to be regarded as a safety hazard, and the familiar grey colour in town and country-side constituted a very definite public nuisance."[47] Townspeople may not have understood the severity of the risk this dust presented to them, but local complaints indicated to the company that dust and asbestos-related disease was becoming a community-wide issue, not one contained to the mine or mill. To address the problem, JM spent $135,000 and five months build-ing a new Cottrell Precipitation Plant designed to reduce dust both in the factory and outside it. This reduced the ambient dust produced by the mill by a fifth, but this still meant that 10 tons of dust were released into the air of Asbestos each day.[48] Dust remained a fact of life in the com-munity in the first half of the twentieth century.

Canadian JM president H.K. Sherry received letters from Asbestos town council thanking him for the improvements made in reducing the amount of fibre hovering over the community and for his commitment to beautifying the town.[49] The community accepted some dust, partly because they trusted JM would not expose them to harm. This local belief was linked to the installation of new, technologically advanced equipment at the C-JM Hospital in Asbestos, such as state of the art X-ray machines, designed to "take hazards out of industry."[50] The hospital was for the entire community, and JM officials stated that "government authorities have expressed interest in the discovery that workers here show remarkable freedom from dust diseases."[51] The people of Asbestos appeared to be the healthiest, most monitored resource workers in the province. With this positive image surrounding the company and the community, JM once again asked Dr. Stevenson for a public assessment of his patients.

Stevenson produced a full report on the health of Jeffrey Mine workers in 1940. He began by once again stating that asbestosis was a misunderstood disease and "the victim of a great many reports." Stevenson continued to assert that asbestosis was not a severe disease, and even if it was, "in this country [it] is not the serious hazard to labor that it was a few years ago believed to be."[52]

Although the symptoms and significance of asbestosis were debated in the international medical community, Stevenson compiled a list of nine generally agreed-on indications of the disease:

1 Dyspnoea [painful breathlessness], the most common, but cannot be noticed except following violent exercise, such as stepping up out of a chair 25 times in 30 seconds;
2 Cough;
3 Cyanosis (late) [unoxygenated blood, poor circulation, blue colouration of the skin];
4 Clubbed finger nails (late);
5 Spitting of blood;
6 Loss of weight and emaciation;
7 Anorexia. When a man cannot eat it is time to stop work;
8 Poor chest expansion;
9 Substernal pain.[53]

By discussing these symptoms, Stevenson acknowledged, but did not address, the pain that some of the workers at the Jeffrey Mine experienced.

While not all of these symptoms occurred at once, and many could be signs of other diseases such as tuberculosis, or simply of poor physical fitness, this list demonstrated JM's willingness to push employees to their bodily limits, as well as the medical profession's lack of compassion and its desire to serve the industry, not the sick. These symptoms also help advance our understanding of what some people in Asbestos experienced.

Townspeople did not need a doctor to tell them that turning blue and coughing up blood meant they were sick. It did not take medical training to connect often painful symptoms to the jobs these men performed at the Jeffrey Mine. The people of Asbestos experienced these symptoms. They continued to refuse to wear respirators while at work, and they did not lobby for better health measures at the mine. JM's suppression of medical evidence clearly affected workers' calculations of the risks they faced. However, the fact that workers remained at the mine despite clogged respirator filters and painful respiratory symptoms indicates that they accepted a degree of bodily risk in exchange for a steady job and a prosperous community.

Reporting on the health of 507 employees who had worked at the Jeffrey Mine for more than ten years (the minimum believed to be required before asbestosis occurred), Stevenson found 17 with early asbestosis, 5 with moderate asbestosis, and none with advanced asbestosis.[54] As low as these figures were (5 percent), Stevenson was quick to point out that they were "arrived at by taking results of Stereoscope examinations only" and that "when these cases are studied from a case history and physical examination standpoint, our percentage of those suffering from Asbestosis [sic] is exactly zero. If we used all of our employees in making these [original] figures, the percentages would be about three times smaller."[55] Stevenson's conclusions suggested that asbestosis was not a problem at the Jeffrey Mine and challenged the views several medical experts held from beyond the community. He seems simply to have been unwilling to believe asbestosis was a problem in Asbestos.

While Stevenson gave a detailed review of the symptoms of asbestosis, he also highlighted some of the customs of the community. Like all JM towns, Asbestos had a Quarter Century Club to recognize those who had worked twenty-five years for the company. "A good percentage of these oldsters," observed Stevenson, "are still doing as hard manual labor as they ever did, and with no more sign of fatigue than any other men of similar age."[56] Although it is likely that local men worked so late into their lives because they needed to support their families, the company's goal was to portray them as tough, healthy, and happy individuals. Stevenson also mentioned the JM employees who had died since 1929: "I have investigated the cause of death in all these cases, and not one of them have died of a lung affection [sic] … Of those living, there is not one that displays the classical signs of Asbestosis [sic]."[57] Once again, Stevenson's conclusions were misleading. He did not perform any autopsies. The exterior physical indicators he relied on for diagnosis were similar to those for a number of other diseases. Furthermore, as a JM spokesperson, he had a vested interest in denying any occurrence of serious health problems in Asbestos.

At the beginning of his report, Stevenson attributed the confusion over asbestosis to the lack of human remains to study,[58] ignoring the fact that he was the doctor in a community that was built around the asbestos industry. He had bodies available. Although he admitted that autopsies were the one conclusive way to determine whether an employee had suffered from asbestosis, he reported that "we have never had reason to have autopsies on our men, owing to the absence of symptons [sic] suggesting Asbestosis [sic]."[59] Rather than fully investigating the effects of asbestos, Stevenson skimmed the surface of signs and symptoms without questioning them.

The people of Asbestos knew that many of them were becoming painfully ill after working at the Jeffrey Mine. Stevenson's assurances that they were healthy, or that their illnesses were caused by other factors, convinced them that the bodily knowledge they possessed through their own suffering was wrong. It is likely that at least twenty-two Jeffrey Mine workers had asbestosis in 1940, but Stevenson's influence, and their complete reliance on the mine for employment, helped ensure that JM employees did not file any complaints against the company. Nor did they lobby for a safer work environment.

Officials at the British manufacturing firm Turner and Newall remained unconvinced by Stevenson's report. Showing a lack of respect for his medical authority, company man F. Bussy wrote to Turner and Newall that "Dr. Stevenson has obviously had but little experience of post-mortem examinations and we shall therefore have to be guided more by men who have the opportunity of many such examinations. I cannot but feel that with their experience of known cases if our Medical Board were to examine the 507 men mentioned there would be more cases to report."[60]

As a company doctor who did not perform the most basic examinations to trace the progression of disease, and who did not publish the results of his studies in medical journals, Stevenson held very little authority outside the community of Asbestos. By sharp contrast, some British and American medical professionals were particularly concerned about industrial health problems like asbestosis and were devoting entire studies to autopsy results. But the authority his profession lent him meant that Stevenson remained effective closer to home. After his report was submitted to the Quebec government, asbestosis was removed from its list of industrial diseases; even the workers' association accepted the decision.[61] Because of his authoritative role when it came to the health of the workers at Asbestos, Stevenson was kept on retainer by JM after he retired in 1945, "due to the number of asbestosis cases that will come up for consideration in the next few years."[62] Soon after, he was elected mayor of the neighbouring community of Danville.

"A SITUATION IS DEVELOPING WITH THE MINERS IN QUEBEC": 1940–49

Stevenson's 1940 report emerged as both the Canadian Medical Association and L'Association des Médecins de Langue Française du Canada turned their attention to diseases afflicting those engaged in war industries.[63] Neither organization had direct access to Jeffrey Mine workers because JM did not allow outside medical professionals access to employee files, but the severity of asbestos-related disease was increasingly evident throughout the province's asbestos region, at mines JM did not operate.

Medical reports on asbestos-related disease emerging from Laval University studies in Thetford in the 1940s were strong where Stevenson was weak. These reports, which included autopsy photos of diseased lungs, noted how quickly and painfully Thetford asbestos workers died once they arrived at the hospital complaining of difficulty breathing.[64] In the first report on asbestos in *Laval médical*, published in 1941, doctors wrote that asbestosis was a disease the medical community knew little about, but that increased collaboration among those treating the illness would solve this growing problem.[65] Francophone medical professionals were able to publish their findings free of interference, and in this first piece, they expressed their suspicions that those associated with JM were not so free.

The doctors at Laval demonstrated this freedom when publishing on two patients who were in their care for asbestosis.[66] These cases led them to believe that asbestosis was a precursor to lung cancer.[67] In this, their reports differed sharply from those released by JM-funded doctors; however, their findings were in sync with those of Leroy Gardner at Saranac. During his study on the effects of asbestos dust on mice, Gardner "unintentionally" found that the mineral caused lung and organ cancer 81.8 percent of the time.[68] In a letter to Vandiver Brown, Gardner wrote that the

> question of cancer susceptibility now seems more significant than I had previously imagined. I believe I can obtain support for repeating it from the cancer research group. As it will take 2 or 3 years to complete such a study, I believe that it better be omitted from the present report ... The evidence is suggestive but not conclusive that asbestosis may precipitate the development of cancer in susceptible individuals.[69]

If these results were released, the repercussions for JM and the economy of Asbestos would be catastrophic. Furthermore, cancer was not something that Jeffrey Mine workers had considered when evaluating bodily risk in the pit and at the mill. This information had the potential to be explosive in the community and throughout the industry. Gardner never published his findings, and JM claimed that there was no proof the mineral caused cancer. After Gardner's death in 1946 and at JM's urging, Saranac researchers published a heavily edited version of the report in an effort to prove the relative harmlessness of the mineral. Industry leaders had again suppressed knowledge of the effects of asbestos dust, on both the mice in Gardner's lab and the men at the Jeffrey Mine.

Although JM exercised authority over the asbestos studies conducted by Saranac Laboratory researchers, it had no control over the medical professionals at Laval. Francophone doctors in Quebec were somewhat isolated from the rest of the North American medical community because of linguistic boundaries, but they were well aware of the studies on asbestos-related disease written in English. In 1943, Laval's Dr. Louis Rousseau believed that asbestos was unique in the way it affected the human body and in its relatively recent emergence as a subject of medical study.[70] The mineral fascinated these doctors because of their proximity to the asbestos-producing region and because of its unusual pathology, not because they had a financial interest in the results of their studies (as was the case with the Saranac doctors). In Rousseau's view, these edited studies were impeding proper legislation in Quebec and placing the asbestos workers of the province at a disadvantage because they could not review proper, unbiased evidence showing the progression of asbestosis. He also stated that companies like JM, which refused to cooperate with independent studies, were the biggest obstacle to acquiring useful information on the disease.[71]

According to Rousseau, workers did not have the power to lobby for improved health standards in the Quebec asbestos industry, however much they mistrusted the mining companies. One indication of workers' powerlessness manifested itself when Quebec premier Adélard Godbout's new Labour Code, which would have facilitated compensation claims and unemployment insurance, failed to pass in the National Assembly after Godbout lost the 1944 provincial election. Union Nationale leader Maurice Duplessis had been elected in Godbout's place, and he had no intention of updating the province's labour laws, especially if they infringed on corporate rights. As far as Duplessis was concerned, companies needed the freedom to act in ways they felt were best for business without worrying about government intervention. Disease legislation stalled.

The growing number of medical reports on asbestos-related disease in *Laval medical*,[72] combined with Gardner's discovery that the mineral caused high rates of cancer in mice, encouraged JM to conduct further studies on its workers in Asbestos. In May 1944, Gardner wrote to Stevenson asking that he be able to review the X-ray films of Jeffrey Mine workers because the population's occurrence of asbestosis was so disproportionately low compared to what had been found in JM's American factories. Although Gardner was given permission to see the X-rays on his visit to Asbestos, C-JM President H.K. Sherry made it clear to Stevenson that "our main interest should be in any favorable findings" that resulted from Gardner's examination of the films.[73]

Fortunately for the company, Gardner confirmed Stevenson's findings. After examining between two and three hundred X-rays with a New York State Department of Health official, Gardner found only two possible cases of "questionable first degree asbestosis."[74] But Gardner had not asked why he had been given only a selection of old films to study, chosen by Stevenson himself. The two cases of possible asbestosis could have been from many years prior and could have turned into lung cancer or premature death by 1944, but Gardner did not follow up on them. The workers at the Jeffrey Mine were not disease-free, but Stevenson's selective approach to choosing films for Gardner to study made it appear as though they were.

Soon after Gardner's 1944 visit, JM and its workers signed a new collective agreement. The union demanded for the first time that a "dust clause" be included in the contract. Its version of it stated as follows: "The Company will take necessary steps to eliminate as much as possible the dust in its operations."[75] C-JM official G.K. Foster insisted that the dust clause be accepted only if absolutely necessary and only if rephrased to read: "The Company recognizes the desirability of progressive improvement in the alleviation of any nuisance arising from the existence of dust in its operations, and will continue to pursue its policy of adopting such measures as it may from time to time deem to be practical, having in view the accomplishment of that objective."[76] The company's alteration amounted to vague allusions to dust control rather than an actual dust clause, but the workers accepted it.

While the company and the union were negotiating the dust clause, JM funded a report on a forgotten segment of the Jeffrey Mine workforce: women. Company doctors acknowledged that most cases of asbestosis were found among its mill workers, but they never mentioned the women who made up 25 percent of the workforce there during the war.[77] In August 1944, JM official Joan Ross examined the female workers at the Jeffrey Mine. She noted that the Textile Department had the worst dust problem and the highest absentee rate in the entire factory, so it should have been studied in the past. Ross attributed the frequent absence of female employees at Asbestos to "dust and bad ventilation, fatigue, and higher absentee rate among women in general."[78] Ross also noted that the "situation has become a topic of conversation throughout the entire community and is a serious detriment to the reputation of the company."[79] The local population seemed to understand risk as pertaining only to male employees. Women were still to be protected from the adverse effects of industrializing the land.

Gendered perceptions of who could be exposed to industrial risk and disease were common in the nineteenth and early twentieth centuries. Because of their perception that mining was male-dominated, JM officials and company doctors had previously ignored the health of female employees. Stevenson felt it was acceptable to move a sick male employee from the mill to another part of JM operations; women could not be sacrificed to the industrial machine or transferred to a job in the mine. They were confined to the dusty Textile Department. Asbestos dust was not supposed to harm wives and daughters, and when it did, townspeople complained. Later that year, the province recommended that improvements be made to control dust at the mill,[80] but these suggestions were not mandatory because of the Duplessis government's unwillingness to infringe on the rights of companies operating in Quebec. The care of female employees at the Jeffrey Mine had to be negotiated between the workers and JM, and the company would not admit they were at risk.

The Duplessis government was not worried about asbestos dust, but the researchers at Laval were, and so were a growing number of international medical professionals, who were making it a primary concern. In 1946, Rousseau again expressed his frustration over the lack of commitment to researching asbestos-related disease in Quebec, which provided 75 percent of the global supply of the mineral. He also expressed dismay that silicosis was well-studied while asbestosis was neglected. He believed that asbestosis was a unique disease that required further study because of its severity. He called for a collaborative study free from the politics and interests of asbestos-producing companies.[81]

Rousseau referred not only to Stevenson's work but also to Gardner's unreleased report, which had been greatly anticipated by the medical community. After Gardner's death, JM released an edited portion of his unfinished report, which stated that the mineral was inert. Rousseau found this impossible to believe. In 1947, Vandiver Brown went even further with Gardner's study by requesting that any reference to cancer be deleted. He then wrote to company attorney J.P. Woodard that the discovery of cancer "looks like dynamite."[82]

Gardner's discovery that the mineral caused cancer – a discovery supported by other international studies – threatened to counter JM's claim that Quebec asbestos was safe.[83] In light of this, company officials went on the offensive against reports emerging from Laval by preparing findings of their own, stating there was "a need to complete Gardner's report before French Canadian researchers elect to write something themselves."[84] Researchers at Laval were convinced that asbestos dust was increasing death rates in the region's mining towns, but the workers at the Jeffrey Mine had not been included in their studies, and they found no further traces of cancer during their autopsies of Thetford employees.[85] It appeared that the results of Gardner's study had been successfully contained, and to ensure it stayed that way, JM installed a new doctor at Asbestos after Stevenson retired.

Dr. Kenneth Smith had worked for JM before moving to Asbestos. He understood what the company expected of him, but he was not always comfortable with this role. One of his first actions was to remove employee Alexandre Bourassa to a less dusty area of the mill. Although Bourassa was only thirty-five years old and did not appear sick, he had worked in the mill for twenty years, and Smith believed that "should he continue to work in the dust much longer ... we might have another case with a typical X-ray film and typical physical findings of asbestosis."[86] Smith was a different kind of doctor than Stevenson. He took the dangers of Jeffrey Mine asbestos much more seriously than his predecessor, and he thought often about his role in putting workers at risk. It is not clear what employees were told or not told when they were transferred from one part of the mine's operations to another after visiting the doctor, or if they worried about what the move might mean. What *is* clear is that Smith believed the people of Asbestos were at much greater risk of disease than they had been told.

Despite this, Smith helped calm JM's fears over what might be discovered by francophone medical professionals studying Thetford workers. He befriended Dr. Paul Cartier at Thetford and scheduled monthly meetings with him to ensure a "uniformity of procedure and results in the two clinics."[87] Smith was able to convince Cartier to keep Thetford health records from outsiders, and between 1947 and 1949, doctors at Laval had no subjects on which to study the health effects of asbestos. The two doctors became friends, and after the medical records at Thetford were closed, Cartier became Smith's ally and confidant. Smith told Cartier of his frustration at not being free to focus on asbestos-related disease. Forced to address every medical ailment in Asbestos, Smith complained to Cartier, "I cannot do as good a job as you are doing, but that is what [JM] wants."[88] In fact, the company had specifically asked him to prevent knowledge of asbestos-related disease from spreading, especially to union representatives."[89]

In the late 1940s, the Congress of Asbestos Miners, a workers' group based in East Broughton, Quebec, had started to meet every year to lobby for asbestosis awareness and prevention. Workers were becoming increasingly aware of the risks associated with asbestos. Vandiver Brown believed that a "situation is developing with the miners in Quebec." He believed that a severely edited version of Gardner's report, one with every mention of cancer – in mice or men – removed, urgently needed to be published in order to counter "opinions being expressed and conclusions arrived at by Quebec physicians and officials upon the basis of surmise, social ideology, and inadequate information. Time therefore is of the essence."[90]

To help ensure that questions about the health of Jeffrey Mine workers were contained within Asbestos, at the end of 1948, when JM and the workers' union were negotiating another contract, the company opened a hospital equipped with the most advanced X-ray technology. At the opening, McGill University's Dr. Viscan extolled JM for its commitment to the health of its employees.[91] Government officials, company heads, and union leaders also celebrated the new C-JM Hôpital et Clinic, but Smith was not happy. He had asked the company to do something about the dust problem in the mill, advising that "if any dust is raised, I believe that the men should wear respirators."[92] Smith was willing to hide X-ray results from employees and visiting researchers, but he was not content to see Jeffrey Mine workers constantly exposed to a severe health hazard that could be reduced.

Employees had each been issued two respirators, but they often refused to wear them because they clogged so easily and made breathing difficult. Even as their knowledge of asbestosis grew, Jeffrey Mine workers minimized the severity of the risks associated with the mineral and their labour. Company officials believed that the health issue was best addressed by eliminating rather than screening dust, but they were slow to introduce the necessary equipment. Until they did, they had a duty to insist that workers wear respirators. They failed to do so.[93]

Smith was caught in the middle. It worried him that JM employees were refusing to protect themselves, and he warned the company that his role in covering up the negative effects of the mineral could damage the industry. At the same time, he made no effort to increase the number of autopsies performed on Jeffrey Mine employees who had passed away, thereby forsaking the chance to learn more about asbestosis. He thought that more autopsies would result in more successful compensation claims.[94] Even though he worried about his patients' health, Smith was primarily concerned with protecting JM.

Early in 1949, a report by Burton LeDoux, an American investigative journalist of French origin, plunged the Quebec asbestos industry into crisis. LeDoux published his exposé on asbestos-related disease, *L'amiantose à East Broughton: un village de trois mille âmes étouffé dans la poussière*, in pamphlet form and in Montreal's *Le Devoir* in January 1949, just as contract negotiations between JM and the workers at the Jeffrey Mine were reaching a deadlock. The report was written in French, the language of most Jeffrey Mine workers, and its publication in a newspaper rather than in a medical journal carried it to a much wider audience than anything that had come before it.

The first section of the report offered a general account of the industry and the diseases the mineral gave to Quebec workers. LeDoux wrote that workers and the general public needed a much more sophisticated understanding of asbestos-related disease because extraction of the mineral was expanding and Quebec had a monopoly on its supply. He stated that the profits being made by the province's asbestos companies had transformed the region's asbestos-mining communities into concentration camps, and that the fatal illnesses plaguing these towns, in which 30,000 people lived, could have been avoided.[95] In LeDoux's persuasive rhetoric, asbestosis suddenly seemed as threatening as a widespread epidemic.

LeDoux wanted to educate asbestos workers about the effects of the mineral on their bodies. He claimed it took only two to three years for asbestosis to develop in the lungs of workers, both young and old, and that every part of the industry, not just the mills, created dust that was too small for the eye to see. Although LeDoux was not a medical professional, he put names to the symptoms that generations of people in Asbestos had suffered from, while informing them that breathing in even a little bit of asbestos dust could condemn them to death.[96]

LeDoux devoted several pages to explaining what asbestosis was and how it affected the human body. He wrote that asbestos dust acted like a spider spinning a web tighter and tighter around the lungs until breathing was so restricted that you suffocated to death.[97] LeDoux wanted to shake workers out of their acceptance of risk and inspire them to mobilize against the companies exploiting their health and labour. He succeeded in this partly because he did not hide any of the frightening effects of asbestosis – that those affected became less and less capable of breathing in fresh oxygen until, very slowly and painfully, their lungs were destroyed and they died.[98] The graphic language he used to describe the deaths he believed awaited the asbestos workers of Quebec countered the assurances company doctors had given over the years to patients who knew they were not physically well, and who saw their friends and family members dying.

Company doctors had been able to pacify employees, LeDoux wrote, because of the basic human desire to deny the imminence and inevitability of death. Moreover, because asbestosis develops slowly, many sufferers died from other ailments such as pneumonia, tuberculosis, and heart disease. LeDoux also stated that the official figures for asbestosis underestimated the situation because companies and their doctors lied to workers. He provided a list of symptoms by which employees could self-diagnose. These included irritation of the nose, throat, and the upper respiratory tubes, shortness of breath, a wet or dry cough, loss of weight and appetite, physical weakness, and chest pain.[99] He also explained that by the time these symptoms became noticeable, it was already too late to stop the progression of the disease.

LeDoux ended his morbid report on a positive note, writing that "ASBESTOSIS IS INCURABLE, BUT IT CAN BE PREVENTED."[100] Responsibility for prevention lay not with companies or doctors but with the workers themselves. After being provoked to outrage at the idea that simply breathing near any of the Jeffrey Mine's operations could condemn them to death, or at the thought that companies had been lying to them about the state of their health, it was the workers' own fault if they became fatally sick. The local newspaper in Asbestos urged townspeople to read LeDoux's piece, and the union distributed copies of it.[101] In February 1949, just weeks after LeDoux's exposé, Jeffrey Mine workers went on strike, demanding that JM provide better protection against the hazards they now knew asbestos posed to their health.

4

Essential Characteristics,
1918–49

S INCE 1983, THE POPULATION of Asbestos has declined by over 50 percent. In 2006, the community was named one of ten towns in Quebec
that would disappear within a decade. This is what happens when a single-
industry town goes into terminal decline. The mayor of Asbestos in 2006,
Jean-Philippe Bachand, attempted to change the name of the community
to Trois-Lacs or Phoenix in order to attract new industry, in the belief that
"Asbestos as a name doesn't sell."[1] Most townspeople disagreed with
Bachand, so the name remains, while he does not. Town councillor Serge
Boislard, whose father died of asbestos-related disease, contended that
changing the name would only "tell the world that we are ashamed of our
product ... [and it would] be one more nail in our coffin."[2]

Asbestos is now excoriated throughout the world, and the townspeople
of Asbestos now understand that it makes people – including themselves
– sick. Even so, the Jeffrey Mine remains fundamental to their identity.
Over two kilometres wide and deeper than the Eiffel Tower is high, the
pit is where the town has taken root; it is what connects land and people.
By exploring how the people of Asbestos oriented their lives, politics,
economy, and faith around the Jeffrey Mine, this chapter tracks the
development of a local body politic and the ways in which residents formed
identities and loyalties alongside the mine as it grew and changed the
community around them between 1918 and 1949.

As the asbestos industry boomed after 1918, the Quebec government actively promoted British and American investment in this and other natural resource industries in the province. Industry leaders declared the men who worked the Jeffrey Mine between 1914 and 1918 to be heroes, likening them to the soldiers who had fought so well in the war.[3] When JM took full ownership of the Jeffrey mine in 1916, officials were well aware that Asbestos was a single-industry and single-company town, and they began to develop a system of paternalistic company-community relations. Despite these early efforts, workers soon went on strike to assert their own power within the town. The miners at Thetford unionized in 1915; those at Asbestos did not yet rely on a union to give them bargaining strength. The fifty men of Asbestos who went on strike were dynamite handlers who made $3.15 a day and believed they should be making $3.50.[4] After a short, peaceful walkout, the company met the workers' demands.

While the dynamite crew at the Jeffrey Mine was greeting JM with a strike, town council sought a close working relationship with the company by making deals in its favour (see Figure 11). JM vice-president and treasurer J.P. Pearson and JM vice-president C.H. Shoemaker were accepted as voting members of the relatively small council. On June 4, 1919, this council passed Règlement 81, which allowed JM to pay for the installation and maintenance of electricity at the mine and throughout the community. The town would buy electricity purchased by JM from the Shawinigan Water and Power Co. by offering the company a property tax remission.[5] Mayor Victor Dubois was the first in the community to have his home equipped with JM's electricity. Council also reduced the road taxes owed by JM even though the company relied on the roads to move its product out of town.[6]

Corporate and council interests seemed to be natural allies as worker unrest increased across Quebec and Canada. In 1919, there were at least 68 strikes in Montreal and 210 throughout Canada.[7] The Communist Party of Quebec was formed in Montreal in May 1919. The Winnipeg General Strike of May and June 1919 worried capitalist interests across the country. JM needed allies to maintain control over its workforce at the Jeffrey Mine, and the town council seemed willing to help.

In October 1919, Jeffrey Mine workers unionized, joining l'Union ouvrière Catholique du Québec (Catholic Workers Union; CWU). Sherbrooke's *La Tribune* attributed this step to the recognition that there was strength in numbers and that it was necessary to improve wages and

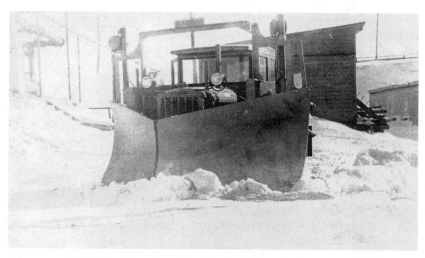

FIGURE 11   Johns-Manville snowplough clearing the streets of Asbestos, 1929–30
Source: WG Clark Fonds, ETRC

working conditions.[8] The CWU drew its strength from outside Montreal, from workers who were averse to radical international unions.[9] The union restricted membership to Roman Catholics, but this was not a major issue in Asbestos, where only 15 percent of the population was not French Catholic (and most of those were JM officials). This was in sharp contrast to other parts in the region, including Shipton Township as a whole, which was 38 percent anglophone, and Sherbrooke, the principal town in the Eastern Townships, which was 29 percent anglophone.[10] The community of Asbestos was divided along linguistic and class lines – a francophone majority made up the bulk of workers; a smaller anglophone faction ran JM. The company resisted the idea of outside union officials influencing its workforce, and it refused to recognize the union for decades after workers joined it.[11]

By the end of 1920, asbestos was crucial to the rebuilding of Europe's cities. This stimulated production at the Jeffrey Mine despite a new US tariff on all manufactured asbestos goods, in response to which Quebec imposed its own 5 percent tax on asbestos exports.[12] Unfazed by the US tariff and the Quebec tax, JM announced in June 1921 that it would be opening a manufacturing plant in the community to produce wool rock for furnaces and asbestos-based textiles.

The new manufacturing plant increased local employment, but international demand began to decline as the postwar boom dissipated. Wages and shifts were reduced throughout Quebec's mining communities, one-quarter of unionized workers in the province were out of work, and the *Canadian Mining Journal*'s hopes expressed late in January 1921, that "a brilliant page of History is about to be unrolled in this Dominion," had seemingly been reduced to ashes by midsummer.[13]

Between 1914 and 1921, the Catholic union movement in Quebec had grown sixfold and had united itself under the Confédération des travailleurs catholiques du Canada (CTCC).[14] By 1922, the CTCC represented 96 unions and 26,000 workers. Both the Church and the provincial government approved of the organization. This gave the CTCC strength, but its leaders were not interested in using it. At its inception, the CTCC was a conservative organization that regarded labour issues as moral ones and that adhered to the social doctrine of the Catholic Church.[15] This approach was based on the *Rerum Novarum*, an encyclical released by Pope Leo XIII in 1891 that encouraged the formation of doctrine-abiding unions by workers who were taught that eventually, the meek would inherit the earth. The existence, and indeed the strength of the CTCC, the largest labour organization in Canada based on cultural and religious values, indicates how deeply the Catholic Church permeated the lives of Québécois in the 1920s. Because of its exclusive membership requirements, the CTCC tended to pit French Canadian workers against foreign, anglophone, and Protestant officials operating companies in Quebec (see Figure 12).

In the economic crisis of the early 1920s, Jeffrey Mine workers deemed employment more important than union solidarity. The company had cut their wages, and they knew other workers would take their places if given the chance, so the workers in Asbestos chose not to push JM to recognize their union.[16] By contrast, the asbestos miners in nearby Thetford were becoming increasingly radicalized by the industrial downturn, and went on strike twice in 1923 without the consent of their union, using guns and dynamite to push their case.[17]

GROWING PAINS: 1923–37

To help stimulate production during the economic slump of the early 1920s, JM constructed its new manufacturing plant, hired more employees, and made a new partnership with the Phillip Carey Manufacturing Co., another US-based company specializing in asbestos products. In 1924, the two companies bought a factory in Lennoxville, Quebec, to produce asbestos paper with fibre extracted from the Jeffrey Mine.[18] As economic

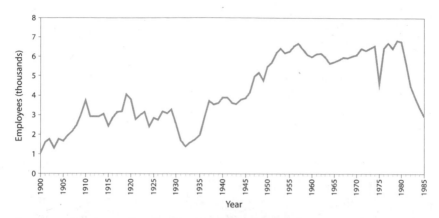

FIGURE 12   Number employed in Quebec's asbestos industry, 1900–85
Source: Data provided by the Province of Quebec (http://www.mern.gouv.qc.ca/mines/
desminesetdeshommes/index.jsp#annexe), compiled by Marc Vallières

expansion continued, the J.P. Morgan Co. bought over half the company's
shares and financially supported JM's industrial ambitions.

Partnerships like these helped to bring Asbestos out of its economic
downturn. Meanwhile, the Asbestos town council further solidified its
relationship with JM. Echoing the doctrine of the CTCC, council agreed
that it was in the best interests of the community to cooperate with JM.[19]
There seemed to be only two factions in Asbestos – the company and
everyone else – and council wanted relations to be harmonious. Optimistic,
JM constructed a Canadian headquarters in Montreal in 1927, and town
council extended its electricity contract for ten more years. In return, JM
received a 45 percent reduction in municipal taxes for land the company
held. Council sacrificed a significant portion of its tax revenue to maintain
good relations: the company paid just over $500 in taxes in 1927, much
less than it owed as the town's largest landholder.[20]

Despite the good relationship being nurtured between town council
and JM, the community was wary of changes. In particular, the local
people were suspicious of newcomers, who were being drawn to Asbestos
by the growing demand for labour at the Jeffrey Mine. Council moved to
charge residents who had lived in Asbestos for less than a year extra municipal taxes, defining them in Règlement 163 as "strangers."[21] In this way,
council was partly compensated for the reduced taxes paid by JM. Clearly,
the community had become adverse to outsiders.

JM was aware of these local concerns but was much more focused on
its international ambitions. By the mid-1920s, the seven asbestos producers

around Thetford had united under the Asbestos Corporation in an act of "patriotic self-preservation" to control wages and prices.[22] JM officials chose not to join it. Although it would still have to abide by US antitrust laws, JM instead joined an international cartel that would be an asbestos "League of Nations," with America's Phillip Carey, Britain's Turner and Newall, and Austria's Eternit.[23] The Asbestos Corporation might have power in Quebec, but through this global alliance, JM now had international influence and was quickly informed of the latest mining technologies and new markets, which further added to the success of the Jeffrey Mine. This success was halted, however, by the Great Depression.

The early 1930s were devastating for Asbestos, as they were to Canada and much of the world. French Canadian organizations such as L'Action française and Les Canadiens français demanded that the government and economists fix the situation. They believed that the economy would have been more robust had it been controlled by people from the province rather than by international firms. As one of those international firms, JM was affected by the changes the Depression brought to the community. With more and more citizens unable to afford electricity, the town suspended its contract with JM, and the company was required to pay the full tax on its land. To go from paying just over $500 in taxes in 1927 to $16,689.86 in 1932[24] was a financial blow to the company, which was already suffering from the global economic downturn. JM officials cited it as one reason they were forced to close the Jeffrey Mine from May 1932 to April 1933.

The closure made life difficult for the community. Many residents had few savings and had to muster a great deal of humility as they turned to town council for aid. At the end of 1933, council applied to the provincially managed Secours-Direct for $800 to help feed thirty local families and clothe and shelter forty-one more.[25] That seventy-one families were in need of aid even after JM resumed operations at the Jeffrey Mine demonstrates the extent to which a year's worth of lost wages had affected the people of Asbestos. Requests for provincial money would continue throughout the Depression.

The process of distributing aid was entirely open. Anyone who asked for financial help from the town was listed in the minutes. Their apparent need was then discussed and voted on by council, and if they received aid, the amount was made public. A single worker who would have made over $3.00 a day at the mine in the 1920s received $1.25 in aid each week during the Depression. Married couples received $1.60 per week,[26] and additional sums were paid for children: $2.00 for one child, $2.20 for two,

$7.20 for fourteen. These were small sums compared with the average household earnings during the boom years.

JM paid its full amount of municipal tax throughout the Depression and accounted for 70 percent of the town's income.[27] After the 1932–33 closure, JM rehired many local employees but operated shortened shifts and was idle on Sundays for the next few years. In July 1934, the town council voted to encourage other industries to come to the community on the grounds that not everyone in Asbestos had the ability to work at the Jeffrey Mine and that the town needed industries that could provide employment for young men and women, as well as for older men.[28] This was the first of many times the town expressed its concern about relying on one industry, but no other major industry ever came to Asbestos.

Along with the economic crisis, the Depression era in Quebec saw a conservative movement sweep the province. Maurice Duplessis, leader of the Union Nationale, was first elected premier of Quebec in 1936, and was unsympathetic to the plight of industrial communities like Asbestos.[29] The Depression and Duplessis's new policies renewed an appreciation for unions in the province's resource communities. Left-wing idealists slowly began to infiltrate the Catholic union movement, whose leaders lobbied workers in the industries of the greatest importance to the province.[30] The union in Asbestos, still ignored by JM, suddenly became energized under the activist leadership of abbé Aubert, a prominent figure in the region's Catholic network in 1936. The hard years of the Depression and its subsequent relief in 1937, combined with the recent urging of the Catholic union movement, convinced workers to try to gain some control over operations at the Jeffrey Mine and do as they had done when JM first came to Asbestos: go on strike.

The workers' demands in 1937 were simple: a wage increase of 33 percent and recognition of their Catholic union. These demands were given to the company two weeks before the strike; JM VP Shoemaker promised that he would respond by 22 January. When no response came, the workers in the manufacturing plant walked out, followed soon after by the men in the Jeffrey Mine. In all, 1,100 men and 50 women went on strike for eight days.[31]

The *Toronto Clarion* called this "one of the most important strikes in the province" because of the financial value of the asbestos industry.[32] However, the dispute had even greater significance for the strikers. Their labour was pulling JM out of the Depression, and their role in the company's success had to be acknowledged. Despite the economic significance of the industry to the province – and to global markets – workers saw this as a local issue, and they rejected Premier Duplessis's overtures to hold negotiations in Quebec City under government supervision: the strike was to remain in Asbestos.[33]

The workers picketed the mine gates in such great numbers that JM staff could not enter the buildings. When P.P. Bartleman, the official in charge of JM's employment office, rode his horse around the striking workers on the morning of the 26th, the picketing crowd forced him back home. Later that afternoon, Bartleman once again rode around the strikers on his horse, this time pointing his revolver at the crowd and "displaying a spirit of bravado."[34] He was quickly disarmed and taken to the mayor's office, where a committee that included three JM heads publicly banished Bartleman from Asbestos. He was put on a train that night bound for Cornwall, Ontario.

Bartleman had worked in Asbestos for almost a decade, and for an impromptu court to order him out of town signalled both the strength of the workers and the company's commitment to a cooperative spirit within the community. This stood in stark contrast to the failed attempts of the Thetford miners in 1923 to have their assistant manager fired. Two days after Bartleman's banishment, Shoemaker returned to Asbestos to participate in strike negotiations. After a day of stalemate, a group of five hundred striking workers entered the Hotel Iroquois, where negotiations were taking place, grabbed Shoemaker, and led him to city hall, where they ordered him to leave Asbestos. He left town the next morning.[35]

According to the *Sherbrooke Record*, "the vice-president was severely beaten up by a crowd of hoodlums," but several other newspapers reported that neither Bartleman nor Shoemaker was harmed, and Mayor Philippe Roy denied that any violence occurred.[36] The *Record*'s hyperbolic account likely reflected the rising influence in Sherbrooke of an industrial bourgeoisie hostile to an unruly working class.

In an attempt to gloss over any residual negative feelings from the strike, H.K. Sherry took over Shoemaker's position at the Jeffrey Mine. The company soon gave employees the wage increase they had been seeking and formally recognized their union. JM president Lewis H. Brown wrote an open letter to union leader Olive Cyr, stating that "we depend upon you and your organization to keep the peace and maintain order and preserve property at Asbestos."[37] The strike was over. The workers had succeeded in getting rid of two senior officials, and JM had signed its first collective agreement with its Canadian employees and their union.[38]

The company's willingness to cooperate with its workers, and its reluctance to hold those who had accosted Shoemaker accountable, demonstrated

JM's understanding of the need to compromise with the workers in Asbestos. It was also a sign of the changing landscape in the province's labour relations. Newspaper reports detailing local workers' success in redefining industrial relations spread throughout the country. The Duplessis government responded by linking unions to communist groups, most notably with the 1937 Padlock Law, in an attempt to damper their rising support and quell their actions.[39] The Jeffrey Mine workers were unwittingly caught up in these changes, and because of the significance of the industry to the province, they wielded an influence beyond their comprehension.

THE TUG OF WAR: 1937–49

Both workers and corporate leaders were cautious in post-strike Asbestos as they attempted to improve relations. In February 1938, the director of Quebec's Department of Mines, A.O. Dufresne, wrote that JM had received a complaint from francophone workers at the Jeffrey Mine that the managing officials did not understand French, which was the only language the majority of employees spoke. The complainant went on to suggest that JM needed to hire managerial staff who spoke both English and French so that all workers could be understood.[40] The communication problems that arose from this situation were frustrating for both sides, and in response, JM began to hire bilingual men for managerial positions.

JM's management was exclusively anglophone, while almost all Jeffrey Mine employees were francophone and had no opportunity to rise up the company ranks. Recognizing this, JM officials approached the province to ask whether any of "our local boys" were eligible for a government program that helped French Canadians qualify for executive positions by earning a university degree in mining engineering. JM stated that by bringing francophones into the upper ranks of the company, it would help change the almost exclusively anglophone business landscape of Quebec. Because of the significance of the asbestos industry to the province, and because of JM's international influence in the global market for the mineral, the Jeffrey Mine was a key location in terms of making dramatic changes in resource management and industrial relations. If an internationally renowned company like JM started employing local French Canadians in managerial roles, other resource industries in Quebec could be pressured to follow suit. This was an important development in how JM managed local relations in Asbestos, whether officials were sincere in their ambitions or not.

JM's apparent sincerity with this initiative was perhaps linked to its paternalistic management of the community as a whole. By placing local men in managerial roles, it might positively influence labour relations. Furthermore, the company would be broadening its influence while quelling the linguistic divisions it had created in the town. In 1938, JM introduced the bilingual *Johns-Manville Photo*, a monthly circular that featured photographs of employees and their families at the mine and at home. Asbestos did not have a local paper, and the circular's first issue explained that while newspapers from outside the community were helpful, "there are always a lot of things going on in the Canadian Johns-Manville organization which are of particular interest to the people here ... which are not carried by the daily newspapers because they are not of general interest outside this community."[41]

The circular was an attempt at community building, but it also amounted to more paternalism: by controlling the information distributed to townspeople through this monthly, the company was shaping the local news they were exposed to and how they would perceive it. JM also used the circular to encourage subtle changes in its employees' behaviour. When company officials noticed that some of its workers were wasting material in the mining and milling process, they explained the problem as a household issue in the *Johns-Manville Photo*:

> If your wife ... were to burn the meat and spill half the potatoes on the floor, you probably would charge it up to bad luck ... But, if this continued to happen every few days and you had to spend a lot more money for supplies just to make sure that there would be enough ... then you'd try to do something to cut down on the waste ... Of course, you could "Fire" your wife. But good wives are hard to find these days and, besides if you did that, there wouldn't be ANYTHING to eat.[42]

The company went on to explain that the same was true for wasting material at the Jeffrey Mine, which cost JM – the head of the household – a significant amount of money it could have spent on higher wages.

Continuing the pattern of paternalistic community building, JM hosted an "open house" at the Jeffrey Mine in 1940 so that townspeople could see "how their husbands, fathers, brothers and sisters turned out the products which have made the name Johns-Manville world famous."[43] This, of course, overlooked the fact that the people of Asbestos were intimately aware of the work at the Jeffrey Mine, through the labour they did each day, the sounds they constantly heard, and the dust they could not avoid coming into contact with throughout the town. The absence of mothers from this list is also significant. Both married and unmarried women worked at the Jeffrey Mine's Textile Department even though conservative Quebec society discouraged this practice in the belief that a woman's place was in the home raising children. Furthermore, the Jeffrey Mine was often celebrated in *Johns-Manville Photo* as the location where young "Asbestos beauties" would find husbands, but they were expected to stop working once they did, despite the financial contribution two incomes would bring to a growing family. The open house was deemed a success in *Johns-Manville Photo*, but what was really a success in Asbestos was JM's paternalistic shaping of the community and its identity.

Gendered expectations for the Jeffrey Mine workforce were revised by the rising product and labour demands of the Second World War. The federal government contracted JM to equip the Canadian Army with fireproof material. In 1940, this included more than $50,000 for firefighting equipment, building supplies, and asbestos fabric to make fireproof uniforms.[44] Also, the US Army and Navy Munitions Board had asbestos on its "critical minerals" list and was prepared to protect its Canadian suppliers by invasion if enemy powers took control of the mines.[45] Canada was industrializing rapidly, and the asbestos industry was a major part of this change. The people of Asbestos drew a sense of importance from the centrality of the Jeffrey Mine to the war effort. Most of the eligible men in Asbestos chose to stay with the mine rather than enlist in the military to fight another British war.[46]

The Second World War was a time of great change in Quebec. For example, the Church's hold on the union movement was shaken by the province's massive industrialization and urbanization during the war years. Secular labour leaders quickly emerged in the province. Union membership grew across Canada during the war until by 1943, one in three union members was on strike at the same time. In Quebec, where the wartime economy was booming, there were 135 strikes in 1942 alone.[47] Despite this mass organization, there was no unrest in Asbestos. The most collectivist activity that occurred in the community was when local citizens founded "Chez Nous Ideal" in 1942.

The aim of this group was to have community members (i.e., not JM) construct houses for townspeople, to promote home ownership, and to reduce dependence on the company for rental accommodation. Although JM had been trying to strengthen its relationship with employees since the 1937 strike, Chez Nous Ideal indicated that the people of Asbestos were growing more concerned about their personal futures and becoming less reliant on the company in the process. Home ownership slowly changed how the community functioned. It also spoke to a growing sense of place in Asbestos – in boom-and-bust resource communities, it makes sense to rent accommodation, whereas home ownership implies both stability and confidence in continued industrial success.

Although the clergy, JM, and the Quebec government feared that strikes and "chez nous" housing organizations meant that the townspeople were becoming increasingly distanced from the company's paternalistic methods, Asbestos was not becoming radicalized in the years following the Depression. In 1938 the community once again voted to continue the prohibition of alcohol within town boundaries. The workers, described by JM as an "industrial army," also successfully lobbied to cancel shifts on Sundays, a major coup, considering the rising demand for the mineral during the war.[48] Furthermore, the new local newspaper preached the importance of women staying at home with their children, in the belief that mothers working industrial jobs were a direct cause of juvenile crime.[49] The maintenance of conservative values was not limited to Asbestos. In 1944, Duplessis and his Union Nationale government were re-elected after a brief Liberal interlude. Asbestos supported this conservative party even though Duplessis's anti-union policies worried labour leaders.[50] In 1944, Duplessis passed the Labour Relations Act, which gave the government the power to recognize or de-accredit unions and to supervise collective bargaining.

Union sympathizers viewed the Labour Relations Act as an open attack on industrial workers and as a reflection of the government's denial of how greatly the province was being transformed by the Second World War.[51] In response to Duplessis's labour policies and the changes the labour movement had experienced during the war, CTCC members elected social activist Gérard Picard as their new president. His election coincided with the gradual abandonment of the union's policy of cooperation with employers, to focus instead on economic democracy. No longer concerned with the good faith of companies, the post-war CTCC focused on changing how industry was run in the province.

The war transformed industrial society and how workers organized in Quebec. In Asbestos, Jeffrey Mine workers began a series of short labour disputes that would last for years. The first of these occurred even before the end of the war, on March 22, 1945, when the men who had been hired to sink the shaft mines beside rue Bourbeau went on strike. Eighteen of the thirty-four shaft sinkers struck, but they were subcontracted workers and were not represented by the union. They demanded higher wages and more reasonable expectations for production, claiming that the footage expected of them each day was almost impossible to reach. JM disagreed, and the demands were refused. Only two of the striking shaft sinkers returned to the job, with local men replacing the other sixteen "as fast as they [could] be located."[52]

That strike failed, but more labour disputes erupted, although never again without a union. These conflicts indicate that the workforce in Asbestos was becoming more and more militant. A review of the major issues in these earlier strikes suggests how local this working-class agitation was. It also indicates that JM was willing to accommodate its employees' demands in order to ensure the smooth functioning of the Jeffrey Mine and the community.

In November 1945, three hundred men and sixty women, all union members working the midnight to 8 a.m. shift at the manufacturing plant, went on a short wildcat strike.[53] The union members complained that non-unionized employees were reaping the benefits won from their labour disputes without paying into the union or standing alongside their fellow workers. The non-unionized Jeffrey Mine employees felt that unionized workers were slowing production by going on strike with outrageous demands. Ontario had addressed this problem the same year with Justice Ivan Rand's ruling on a strike at Ford. The resulting Rand Formula declared that all employees had to pay union dues, although they would not be forced to join the union. This formula was initially enacted only by Ontario, but unions throughout Canada saw it as an ideal goal to achieve.

In January 1946, dissatisfaction with their foreman triggered a short wildcat strike by 150 railway employees.[54] They claimed that he was prone to "swearing when giving orders to his men, being unnecessarily rough at work, expecting too much to be done, [and was] unqualified for the job."[55] The foreman was refused promotion when JM investigated the accusations and found them to be true.

Generally, the union was wary of pushing JM too far during this period. When thirty-six diggers working inside the Jeffrey Mine went on a wildcat strike in May 1946 that prevented 175 pit employees from doing their jobs because they depended on the striking men, the union ordered them back to work.[56] The dispute lasted only one hour, and both JM and the union rejected the wage increase the diggers had demanded. That the strike had been stymied by their own union was a blow to Jeffrey Mine workers; it also demonstrated that even with social activist Picard as the new president, the CTCC was still less militant than other unions in the province. As a consequence, the CTCC's postwar membership fell to 24.2 percent of Quebec's union membership, down from 37 percent in 1936.

Unlike the CTCC, the asbestos industry was thriving in the postwar period. In JM's annual report for 1948, the company acknowledged that "there is almost no field of human endeavour in which, at some stage or another, some JM product does not play a part."[57] This all-pervasiveness of the mineral added to the growing confidence of Quebec's asbestos miners, and they wanted to strengthen their positions, as well as the union's. Without their labour, extraction levels would surely drop, putting a halt to the industry's rising profits, but without strong unions, their ability to gain higher wages and better health regulations was limited. At the end of 1947, the province's asbestos workers had successfully lobbied their companies to establish uniform contract and negotiation procedures throughout Quebec's asbestos industry. The Rand Formula became the next top demand among asbestos workers, but companies were more reluctant to agree to this measure, which would radically change labour organization and collective bargaining in the industry.[58]

These strikes threatened the traditional paternalistic relationship in Asbestos. In an attempt to reverse this tide, JM officials from New York visited the town in April 1948 to discuss various ideas such as improving public relations through a weekly radio show, circulating information pamphlets more widely, and forging closer ties with the local newspaper.[59] The company wanted to avoid a major confrontation with its workers. But after the visit, Quebec's labour minister, Antonio Barrette, wrote to the Commission des relations ouvrières and the provincial arbitrator that there was "a problem brewing" in Asbestos.[60] Seventy-two Jeffrey Mine employees were upset with JM for introducing new shovels in the pit that required fewer men to work them.

There were signs of rising worker frustration. The local newspaper reported that there had been incidents of sabotage at the Jeffrey Mine. Shift managers had discovered foreign objects in the raw asbestos being milled, which broke processing machines and damaged JM's reputation when tainted bags of the mineral were sold.[61] According to the company, these incidents constituted negligence, not malicious sabotage; the townspeople were shocked that workers had been accused. Good relations between JM and its employees were crumbling. From January to April 1948, Jeffrey Mine workers made more than ninety-two suggestions for workplace reforms – more than the entire number in 1947.[62] When JM refused a request

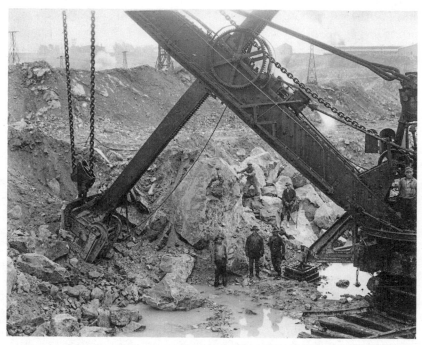

FIGURE 13　Shovels in the Jeffrey Mine, 1930s–40s
Source: WG Clark Fonds, ETRC

that there be no job losses due to the introduction of new shovels, workers became even more agitated.

The new technology JM planned to introduce to the Jeffrey Mine (see Figure 13) would significantly increase extraction levels while reducing employment in the pit by 40 percent. In response to this possibility, the provincial arbitration board reported that there was a "serious threat of strike" if it were to happen.[63] JM did not heed the warning.

The union wanted fixed salaries included in the new collective agreement. This would ensure job stability if the new technologies being introduced made employees redundant. This goal became even more important after JM announced that the Wool Rock Department at the factory would be closed in July and moved to Toronto, where furnace products could be manufactured at reduced cost.[64] Workers were angry. They believed that JM had a responsibility to employ the people of Asbestos and not replace them with machines or cheaper labour elsewhere. Local union leader Armand Larivée warned that if the company did not agree to fixed wages and no staff reductions, there would be trouble during the next contract negotiation period.[65]

Amid all this local turmoil, the people of Asbestos re-elected their mayor, Albert Goudreau, as their MNA in the provincial election of 1948. They were quickly disheartened with his Union Nationale party, however, when the Duplessis government introduced the draft for a new provincial Labour Code, Bill 5. This bill was supposed to bring recommendations and suggestions from employers and employees to the provincial government, but the CTCC rejected it completely, not trusting Duplessis to acknowledge the concerns of workers. This was a sharp departure from the spirit of cooperation preached by the Catholic union before the Second World War. Because of the CTCC's openly hostile rejection of Bill 5, it was withdrawn from the Quebec legislature.[66]

The defeat of Bill 5 was a significant victory for the union movement in Quebec. In January 1949, CTCC President Gérard Picard arrived in Asbestos with newly appointed secretary Jean Marchand to negotiate a new collective agreement with JM that would include salary and job security. The community greeted them with a parade, as if they were war heroes returning from the front. Picard and Marchand gave the local union its own flag, and all the workers at the Jeffrey Mine, and their families, were required to attend a meeting with them on January 14 in the basement of St-Aimé Catholic Church so that they could discuss new contract negotiations.[67]

Of the 2,083 employees at the Jeffrey Mine, 1,733 were directly affected by the negotiations that the CTCC officials were there to settle. Not included in the new contract were employees under the age of sixteen, office staff, and supervisors.[68] The majority of mine employees lived in the community; most of the residents of Asbestos had a direct stake in the mine's operations. The workers had faith in Picard and Marchand, but after only two weeks, union negotiations with JM officials broke down.[69] At the start of February 1949, the community was uncertain what would happen next as a standoff developed between the fundamental factions of the community: the working-class francophone majority; the town council, now allied with the Union Nationale; and the elite anglophone minority that ran the Jeffrey Mine. As the strike of 1949 began, the community of Asbestos found itself confronted by internal and external forces that would bring about radical change during the five months the dispute lasted.

5
Bodies Collide: The Strike of 1949

I N ASBESTOS TODAY, you do not ask lightly about the 1949 strike. A
profoundly local crisis, the strike has become part of Quebec's political
discourse.[1] Those who did not take part in it have romanticized it, overlooking that it temporarily crippled the entire community and forever
changed how power was negotiated at the Jeffrey Mine. Despite the time
that has passed, the animosity between strikers and strikebreakers remains,
and the conflict is not something townspeople are willing to discuss with
outsiders.[2] How the community experienced the strike could not be more
different from how scholars have written about it since. The people of
Asbestos could not keep the political discourse of the province out of the
history of their community, but it was the local experience of the 1949
strike that changed the lives of those who constituted that community, as
concerns over asbestos-related disease were sacrificed for job security.

Just before midnight on February 13, 1949, Jeffrey Mine workers met
in St-Aimé Catholic Church and, against the advice of their union leaders,
voted to strike. A few days later, every other asbestos mining community
in the region except East Broughton followed. Because they did not wait
for the provincial government to establish an arbitration board, the workers
were violating Quebec's Loi des Relations ouvrières. Thus, the strike was
illegal.[3]

The Jeffrey Mine workers went on strike to revise their collective agreement with JM. Their demands turned on three main issues: how land was
used in Asbestos; how asbestos fibres affected workers' health; and how
community decisions and dynamics were negotiated among the working

class, town council, and JM. After Burton LeDoux's 1949 exposé on asbestosis, JM employees no longer trusted the company and refused to return to work until health hazards had been properly addressed and toxic dust had been eliminated. Through the five months of its duration, the strike also revealed a broader struggle in Asbestos – and Quebec – over who would dictate the development of resource communities and industry in the province: the French Canadian working-class majority, or the anglophone managing elite.

"This Strike Won't Last 48 Hours": February to March 1949

February 1949 began unexceptionally. Town council sought a provincial grant to attract new industry and annexed more land on which to build new houses for the growing population. JM paid over $8,000 in municipal taxes, and Dr. Kenneth Smith wrote a report on the need for better dust control measures at the mill. JM also announced to its employees that 1948 was "BIG NEWS!" – the postwar boom had produced record profits for the company.[4] Asbestos workers were well aware of the local role they had played in bringing global economic success to the community through international trade networks. Many of them had been with the company for more than twenty-five years, longer than many of its managers. Despite CTCC secretary Jean Marchand's request that they wait for contract negotiations with JM to address their concerns, they were confident in their ability to achieve contract reform. When the evening shift of February 13 ended at midnight, the Jeffrey Mine went silent as workers walked out. Local police chief Albert Bell allowed the striking workers to use the city hall as their headquarters.[5]

The strikers' major demands were a raise of 15 cents to bring wages to $1.00 an hour, plus five cents more for night shifts (which would cost JM an additional $120,000 each year); job security so that machines would not replace workers; better dust control to prevent asbestosis beyond a vague dust clause; more time off; union input in promotions; and the adoption of the Rand Formula so that 3 percent of the wages of all employees, even non-unionized ones, would have to be paid as union dues. These demands were all similar to those made at some point during previous strikes, but when combined into one overarching dispute, they shook the industry.

JM rejected the Rand Formula, opposed union input on promotions, and refused to admit to a health problem at the Jeffrey Mine. The workers remained resolute, aware that their action would choke the supply of asbestos to most of JM's twenty manufacturing plants. They also forced the three hundred non-unionized employees at the Jeffrey Mine to stop work. Chief Bell reported that the strikers were acting calmly and quietly. When not picketing at the gates of the Jeffrey Mine, they held members-only meetings, which were closed to all but one reporter, Gérard Pelletier, who worked for Montreal's *Le Devoir*. Pelletier was a friend of Marchand, and when he was sent to Asbestos at the start of the conflict, Marchand told him, "if you have your toothbrush, that will be enough. You won't even need your pyjamas; this strike won't last 48 hours."[6] Pelletier would remain in Asbestos for five months. Although he was the only member of the press who stayed in the community for the duration of the conflict, and the only reporter workers allowed into their homes, scholars have never studied Pelletier's reports in depth.[7]

Pelletier spent months getting to know the people involved in the strike and how they interpreted and coped with the changes the conflict had brought to their community. The regional newspaper, Sherbrooke's *La Tribune*, which supported JM, suggested that the workers were bitterly divided over the strike and argued that their wages and health benefits were adequate. *Le Devoir* "not only took the side of the striking workers" but also conducted, according to Pelletier, "a systematic campaign on their behalf throughout the course of the conflict."[8] Pelletier's experiences in Asbestos revealed a strongly conservative and religious populace, not the left-wing, secular idealists they were later described as being. At least once a day, strikers celebrated mass at St-Aimé, and when outsiders arrived with alcohol to raise the spirits of the workers, they were chased out of the dry community. Showing just how nonconfrontational were the early days of the strike, picketers even let some JM employees enter the Jeffrey Mine to pump out the groundwater filling the pit, to avoid damage to equipment.[9]

This changed on February 18, just after the local paper published a message from JM stating that the demands of the workers were unreasonable. Two hundred strikers broke through the mine gates, drove the factory manager and two female office staff from the property, and seized their paycheques from the week before.[10] They would not be paid again for at least five months. The company sent frantic telegrams to Premier Duplessis and Labour Minister Barrette requesting the assistance of Quebec's provincial police, the Sûreté. Portraying a state of anarchy in the town, JM officials showed no hesitation in becoming supplicants of the province:

> When the municipal council is silent can we not count at least on the immediate assistance of the police force of this province ... We have been here more than a half century operating and maintain that our record and our rights call for a measure of protection ... If you ignore further request we feel that any consequence from violence will be your responsibility.[11]

Despite JM's claims, neither Chief Bell nor town council were alarmed by the situation in Asbestos, although four more officers were hired to bring the local police force to eleven men. Workers and local policemen were neighbours and even played cards together at the beginning of the strike. Strikers picketing the gates outside the Jeffrey Mine allowed Bell to pass through in order to make sure the pumps were running properly.[12]

Arguing that the strikers had entered company property forcibly and illegally when they collected their cheques, JM sued the union for $500,000 in damages and filed an injunction to prevent picketing. At 2 a.m. on February 20, sixty provincial policemen arrived in Asbestos. Their presence immediately changed the character of the strike – and the town. Relations between company and community, upper class and working class, anglophone and francophone, shifted radically as JM sought to crush the strike before the workers' health issue became a major cause.

The people of Asbestos saw the presence of the provincial police as an invasion of their community and as an insult to striking workers. Bell told *La Tribune* that "if they come, there will be trouble ... The strikers are peaceful and they have not damaged any property." Pelletier reported that the arrival of the police was "considered in Asbestos as an unjustified gesture of suspicion."[13] Emphasizing the illegality of the strike and sending in the provincial police suggested that JM and the government saw the workers as criminals, which offended the local population. The night the provincial police arrived, seven young strikers followed one of their patrol cars through the streets. They were quickly apprehended after they demanded to know what the police were doing there.[14] Their actions had expressed a certain local confidence, but after several hours of interrogation, the strikers were released, shaken, in tears, and apologizing.

The Asbestos town council had to address the new police presence, especially because the policemen were each paid $50 a week by JM and brought alcohol into town. According to the minutes of a February 21 council meeting, local officials believed there were 150 officers in the community, that they had arrived drunk, and that they had already committed violent, indecent acts likely to provoke rather than prevent trouble.[15] Headlines in leading Toronto newspapers screamed: "Police Drunk, Indecent, Caused First Disorders."[16] Understanding the threat the police posed to community-company relations, council voted unanimously for immediate removal of the force.

In response, the director of the Sûreté, Hilaire Beauregard, issued a statement saying there were only sixty provincial police in Asbestos. Some, he said, had beer with their dinner, but none had time to become drunk.[17] Pelletier contradicted this, saying that many provincial policemen were seen bringing supplies of beer from Danville and Richmond to their temporary barracks in JM's Hotel Iroquois.[18] The provincial police remained in town, escorting office staff through the gates of the Jeffrey Mine, patrolling the streets, and enforcing an evening curfew. The strikers expressed their outrage at a union meeting on February 22, but renewed their commitment to a nonviolent strike. This inspired parish priest and union head Father Louis-Philippe Camirand to poke fun at reports suggesting the people of Asbestos were uncivilized. Much to the delight of his parishioners, he insisted that he was "happy to live amongst such savages."[19] Camirand's support convinced workers that their strike was morally just and encouraged them to remain resolute in their commitment to their demands.

From JM's point of view, council's resolution against the police ignored the real violence of the dispute, which included an illegal strike and the invasion of company property. When rumours began to spread early in March that the company was seeking replacement workers from outside the community, the townspeople deemed apt Pelletier's characterization of JM as the "toughest" of the asbestos companies.[20]

JM denied that it intended to break the strike but warned that a long strike would have far-reaching effects. The company also sent strikers weekly letters urging them to return to work so that negotiations could begin. The letter of February 28 claimed that the union was concealing facts from strikers, and focused on the illegality of the conflict and the damage to Jeffrey Mine equipment the strike had caused.[21] By bypassing the union in this manner and appealing directly to the workers' sense of law, order, and duty, JM was seeking to split the strikers from the union, in the mistaken belief that the employees were less militant than their leaders. The company letter changed nothing.[22]

As the strike continued, and the injunction against picketing at the Jeffrey Mine was extended into April, Mayor Goudreau began to express his fears for the future of Asbestos. In March, he told the press that the local economy was suffering because of the strike, since JM was the community's main employer. Municipal affairs had been frozen by the conflict, with urgent projects being suspended indefinitely.[23] Rumours that the strike might continue for months plagued the community. To address these worries, Marchand and local union head Rodolphe Hamel held a meeting on 6 March solely for the wives of men on strike, with the goal of ensuring that workers had the support of their families.

Pelletier wrote that the hall at St-Aimé was full of young women, old mothers, and the many children whom striking fathers could not look after even though they were not at work. The role reversal – wives and mothers at a union meeting while the striking men of Asbestos remained at home – suggests how much the conflict and the issues it raised were affecting the community. For two hours, the women listened to union representatives speak about the goals of the strike. Their questions addressed worries about the government revoking the union's certification, concerns about the illegality of the strike, fears of what asbestos did to human health, and how their families were to be supported without any wages.[24] After the women left the hall, strikers, both male and female, entered it, "more serious, [and] less light-hearted, after three weeks on strike."[25] Pelletier reported that morale was revived, however, as the meeting turned into a rally for Marchand, whom JM had named the biggest obstacle to a resolution and whom the Quebec government had banned from the negotiating table.[26]

JM sent a second letter to its employees, stressing the illegality of the strike and asserting that Jeffrey Mine jobs were among the safest and best paid in the country.[27] This was the only time JM openly acknowledged the health concerns of its workers, but it did so only to dismiss them and to suggest that workers were overreacting. Once again, JM had failed to recognize the legitimacy of the workers' concerns about their occupational health and job security. This second letter included a ballot that asked workers whether they wanted to end the strike and return to the Jeffrey Mine. Most of the strikers refused to fill it out.[28] Reasons for this refusal include a lack of trust in the company, disbelief that the vote had any validity, and fear of betraying the union by being seen entering JM offices with their ballots.

Undeterred, the company published a full-page advertisement in the local newspaper stating that strikers secretly wanted to return to work, and asserting that each employee lost $7.90 in wages every day and that Asbestos lost $90,000 each week because of the conflict.[29] The loss of wages and JM's continued focus on the strike's illegality did not convince the people of Asbestos to push for an end to the conflict or to ignore the health problems rooted in the Jeffrey Mine. Instead, the ad angered the community. Townspeople accused the editor of the local paper, J. Osias Poirier, of being against the strikers because he so often published JM's opinions. In response, he claimed that union heads ignored his requests for information.[30]

JM's efforts to win over public opinion were weakened by their lodging of the provincial police in employee housing and by the rigidity with which the police applied the law. The police immediately sent local residents to a Sherbrooke jail for any offence, such as driving without a licence. Prior to the strike, misdemeanours like these would have been handled by the local justice system in Asbestos, not the regional centre. The sense that townspeople were being treated as criminals by an outside police force funded by the company created a deep divide between JM and the community.[31]

Tension finally erupted into violence just after 11 p.m. on March 14, when a small group of strikers blew up twenty feet of railway line running between the Jeffrey Mine and the Grand Trunk station at Danville.[32] The attack was a response to rumours that outside strikebreakers were being brought in to work the mine. Blowing up the tracks was a dramatic articulation of how the mine belonged to the people of Asbestos through their labour, their sacrifices, and their history. The night following the explosion on the train tracks, a group of strikers attacked a non-unionized worker, Paul Beauchemin, outside city hall.

Beauchemin had been working at the Jeffrey Mine for only three months and was not on strike. It angered strikers that this relative newcomer continued to earn wages for helping to keep the mill running. They beat him until the provincial police arrived and took him to the JM hospital.[33] By contrast, when striker Edmond Delorme broke his leg attacking a company truck the evening after Beauchemin was assaulted, he was taken to a hospital in Sherbrooke – a reminder to workers of how dependent they were on the company's health facilities.[34]

The union excused the violence done to the tracks and to Beauchemin as a reaction to provocations by the provincial police. But the union's claims were more self-serving than likely. Although strikebreakers had never been used at the Jeffrey Mine, union heads asked town council to refuse "scabs" entry into the town.[35] Employees may have had genuine concerns about outside workers taking their jobs, but council had no power to restrict JM's hiring.

A Moral and Just Strike: March to April 1949

JM responded to the violence by accusing the union – not the strikers – of breaking the law. This was another attempt to drive a wedge between the workers and the CTCC.[36] Advertisements placed in the local newspaper stressed that the company would protect the rights of its employees; it claimed that JM had operated without conflict for more than twelve years, conveniently forgetting the six strikes that had occurred in Asbestos over that time. JM also claimed that the ballots it had sent out the week before showed that 97 percent of strikers secretly wanted to return to work, but as Pelletier pointed out, this statistic was so ridiculous that it became a source of great hilarity (and improved morale) for the strikers.[37] The company had no chance of gaining the support of workers until it addressed issues of land, health, and community. Even Dr. Kenneth Smith believed that JM could not ignore these concerns. He wrote to company officials urging them to stop denying the dangers of asbestos.[38] But this would have amounted to an official acknowledgment that asbestos posed a threat to human health, and the company demurred.

The arrival of a truckload of provisions donated by the people of Sherbrooke on March 18 boosted the spirits of those on strike and made them even more determined to continue the dispute.[39] The company could not starve them back to work, and strikers' worries over how to support their families were eased. Although the donated food boosted community spirit, Asbestos remained bitterly divided along linguistic, class, and religious lines. This divide quickly reached the town's churches. The largely Catholic provincial police heard mass and took communion at JM's Hotel Iroquois, so they were fully removed from the townspeople when not on patrol. The majority of JM officials were Protestant and therefore attended a separate church.

The average citizens in Asbestos revealed which side of the conflict they were on by attending one of two Catholic churches in the community. Local union official Father Camirand gave mass each day at St-Aimé and publicly defended the workers. Father Alphonse Deslandes at St-Isaac-Jogues spoke against the strike, stating it was bad for the families of Asbestos, of whom fifty to sixty would be unable to pay rent by the end of March. In response, several citizens expressed their desire to "kick the priest's [Deslandes'] teeth in."[40]

Tension was especially high in Asbestos because JM had begun to employ strikebreakers to process the fibre that remained at the mill. Anyone who threatened one of these strikebreakers was arrested. On the night of March

22, more than thirty policemen arrived at Roger Beauchemin's home on rue Albert to arrest Émilien Richer. The charge was intimidation against a strikebreaker. When Beauchemin refused to allow the police into his home, they stormed in and dragged him, Roland Paradis, Rosario Bernier, Richer, and his screaming, pregnant wife out into the street.[41] The entire group was then sent to a Sherbrooke jail.

The community was outraged. A local policeman commented that "I never thought I'd meet men who would do such dirty work," and Pelletier reported that the entire community was disgusted by the incident.[42] This disgust extended to JM, and community-company relations deteriorated rapidly. Camirand spoke out against the police, telling the press that "if I was a miner, I'd be on strike myself, given the circumstances, with a peaceful conscience."[43]

On March 24, the company responded to the situation by sending a third letter to its employees. This was also printed in the local paper for the entire community to read. It stated that the strike was not going well, that negotiations had not taken place since early February, that the company was not going to give in to demands, and that it would not fire strikebreakers when the dispute was over.[44] Tired of projecting a friendly image, JM officials were seeking to frighten employees back to work – but they did not shake the strikers' resolve.

Truckloads of food from Sherbrooke and Montreal arrived in Asbestos and helped alleviate some worries about the length of the strike. So too did a financial donation from union members in Shawinigan and the assistance of the Comité de secours. That committee had been established by town council during the Great Depression to help feed local families, and council re-established it in March 1949 in order to pay the grocery accounts of the striking workers on application.[45] Donated food was greatly appreciated by striking workers and their families, but not by local merchants, who were losing valuable customers during the lengthy dispute. These merchants attempted to meet with JM and the union to act as intermediaries and quickly end the strike; both refused the offer.[46]

On March 27, the striking workers feted the arrival of two more truckloads of food from Montreal. The provincial police walked through the streets singing songs of their own during the parade, but there was no reaction from the strikers. This inspired the editor of the local paper to report that calm had settled on Asbestos and that an end to the strike was near. But tension remained, especially between those on strike and the non-unionized JM employees who were not. On March 29, Gérard "Tiny" Newcombe was assaulted outside a company-owned club in Danville by a group of strikers, one of whom was Jean-Noël Hamel, son of local union leader Rodolphe Hamel. Newcombe was taken to JM's hospital in Asbestos; Hamel was arrested. This attack was revenge against Newcombe, who had allegedly beaten a striker outside a club in Richmond the night before. Animosity reigned on both sides of the dispute, and Rodolphe Hamel accused JM of planting spies in the town.[47]

Strikers quickly used the idea of spies to defy the company and the provincial government. When three more truckloads of food arrived in Asbestos from St-Hyacinthe, marchers in the welcome parade carried signs depicting those whom they considered to be the key antagonists in the dispute: C-JM president G.K. Foster, C-JM and QAMA lawyer Yvan Sabourin, and Labour Minister Antonio Barrette. Signs bore the slogans, "No contract, no work," "Our strike is just and moral," and, more mocking, "Long live the provincial police," and "Who blew up the railway?"[48] The workers also handed out fliers to the crowd mocking Tommy Manville, the "asbestos millionaire," for his eight failed marriages, the seventh of which had lasted less than eight hours.

The humour that strikers displayed on their signs revealed an important characteristic of the community: even when a significant portion of the population could not afford to feed their families, a local camaraderie remained. This same spirit was seen when strikers produced a board game resembling Snakes and Ladders that reflected the major issues in the labour dispute. At the top of the ladders were positive things like a growing union membership or a happy family because of fair wages earned. At the bottom were the more negative aspects of the industry: company heads paying for tropical vacations with the money workers earned them, and deaths due to asbestosis – highlighting once again how much health concerns had permeated the community.[49] Proceeds from the sale of the board game went directly to the union.

The Asbestos town council was increasingly concerned about ensuring that the community survived the conflict. JM had paid over $8,000 in municipal taxes in April, but because of the social assistance the town was providing for the workers and their families – $24,729.34 in March alone – Asbestos was rapidly falling into debt. Each week, council paid for up to 2,500 bottles of milk and 4,000 loaves of bread; it had also handed out two hundred sacks of potatoes.[50] By the start of April, the 2,100 employees on strike had passed their seventh week without a paycheque, and while the CTCC had provided $100,000 in strike subsidies, Mayor Goudreau stated that "the loss in wages in Asbestos alone [was] about $800,000 ... [and]

there is a danger of some merchants going bankrupt."[51] The strikers did not want to admit it, but the community was completely dependent on JM.

Yet JM, like so many resource companies, depended on its workers, and the company as a whole was feeling the strike's impact. *La Tribune* reported that many of the company's American processing plants had either shut down or were laying off employees. This included the facility at Manville, New Jersey, where the community depended on processing fibre from the Jeffrey Mine.[52] The same article indicated that the American auto industry was suffering from a lack of supply and that prices for asbestos were higher than they were during the Second World War. To be sure, high prices had sustained the company's profits, which were only beginning to fall.

With profits declining, JM recruited more strikebreakers to process the raw fibre remaining in the mills at the Jeffrey Mine. It also offered workers a raise of 10 cents (rather than the 15 cents being demanded) and the four paid holidays they had asked for. Perhaps sensing the opportunity for more, strikers refused the offer. If anything, JM's sudden willingness to compromise gave strikers more confidence – they took it as a sign that the company was weakening. Besides which, they had not forgotten their demand for better dust control at the Jeffrey Mine. One worker responded to the strikebreakers by telling Pelletier they were welcome "to make a bit of dust."[53]

It is possible that health concerns influenced the company's sudden willingness to compromise. In a letter from JM executive J.P. Woodard to C-JM president G.K. Foster, Woodard detailed Leroy Gardiner's original Saranac study on mice, which showed that even a limited exposure to asbestos dust caused serious lung damage. Woodard encouraged Foster to investigate the level of dust at the Jeffrey Mine to see how dangerous working conditions actually were.[54] The issue of dust raised by the strikers was connected to a much broader health problem within the asbestos industry. JM needed to find a way to address the issue of dust without weakening perceptions that the mineral was safe. Gardiner's study was not published, but the longer that employees were on strike and publicizing the effects of asbestos dust in newspapers like *Le Devoir*, the more likely it was that additional research would be done outside the control of JM.

After the workers rejected JM's offer, the editor of the local newspaper, *L'Asbestos*, felt it was necessary to intervene in the strike. J. Osias Poirier wrote that Asbestos was one of the most important communities in the region, poised to become even greater. He believed that diversification was the key to success but warned that no new industry would come to the community if it gained a reputation for having unruly workers.[55] He urged the strikers to accept the compromises made by JM for the future of the entire town. Poirier's argument had little impact, even though he was correct to emphasize the need for the community to attract new industry. What he failed to consider was that town council had attempted to bring new industry to Asbestos in the past and had failed. Named as it was, and with the massive Jeffrey Mine looming in the centre of it, Asbestos was not much of a draw for other industries. Furthermore, resource communities like Asbestos often fail to diversify, for extraction is the focus of daily operations, and when a booming market is combined with good industrial relations, everyone wants to take part.

Poirier's attempt to address an overarching issue in the community – the lack of industrial diversification – ignored the real crisis on the ground as strikers became increasingly desperate to achieve their aims. This desperation was reflected in the continued attacks on those who continued to work for JM. Just days after Poirier's editorial, strikers threw rocks through the windows of the homes of nine non-unionized Jeffrey Mine workers, allegedly striking Adélard Fortin as well as Ernest Dionne's sleeping baby.[56] More provincial policemen arrived in Asbestos to enforce order against "the terror that reigned" there – although Pelletier wrote for *Le Devoir* that this characterization was a gross exaggeration.[57] The following day, the strikers sent a telegram – addressed with ironic intent to the Minister of Capital – to Labour Minister Antonio Barrette demanding his resignation because he had termed the strike illegal and said the community was in a state of anarchy that went against the doctrine of the Church.[58] Barrette did not reply.

In response to the increased violence, JM went on the offensive once again. To combat the growing press coverage of the workers' concerns about asbestosis, company doctor Kenneth Smith issued a statement claiming that the population of Asbestos was healthy and emphasizing that he, not Burton LeDoux or *Le Devoir*, was the expert on the bodies of those who worked at the Jeffrey Mine. For many reasons, this was an apt implication: it was Smith, not LeDoux, who had examined Jeffrey Mine workers' bodies for years, and LeDoux had never even been to Asbestos. Smith maintained that only two cases of asbestosis had been found in the community in the past fifty years[59] and that studies showed that the air quality in Asbestos was similar to that of any other industrial city in Canada. Smith also claimed, inaccurately, that every JM employee was given a yearly X-ray that was available for anyone to see; in fact, annual exams were running years behind, and nobody outside the company was allowed to see the workers' medical files. Of course, Smith's statement contradicted everything he had confidentially reported to JM and wilfully obscured the health risks associated with asbestos.

Continuing on the offence, JM informed its striking employees that they and their families would soon be removed from company-owned homes. Because rent was taken directly out of wages, it had not been paid since the strike began. JM officials wanted the houses for the three hundred strikebreakers now at the Jeffrey Mine. G.K. Foster wrote to Barrette that "we have felt duty bound to inform the occupants of our dwellings that they must consider resumption of work and understand that we must sooner or later make room for actually [sic] working employees so that we respect the objective for which these houses have been built."[60] Foster's letter portrayed JM as the victim of a negligent working class, which was the only hope the company had of not appearing to be a villain forcing families out of their homes. Evictions would cause problems in Asbestos, where livable space had already been pushed to the town's limits. The population already feared being unable to feed local families. Now they had to worry about housing them, too.

The workers took this new threat especially badly. Not only were their homes and families at risk, they were being threatened by the need to accommodate strikebreakers from outside the community. This filled the strikers with anger. In response, one of them wrote to Prime Minister Louis St-Laurent asking why he was not intervening in the strike and wondering if he cared more about Duplessis's lies than about the plight of the workers who had shaped the economy of Quebec and perhaps even Canada.[61] Father Camirand, who represented one side of the Catholic Church's divided opinion on the conflict, declared that the company and its scabs would have to trample over his dead body to evict the striking workers.[62] Jean Marchand stated that JM never failed to threaten its French Canadian workers, who were so vital to the extraction of one of Quebec's "best natural resources."[63] He also accused the company of treating the working class of Asbestos as slaves to their industrial greed, and emphasized that the asbestos found in the Jeffrey Mine belonged to the people of Quebec, not an American company.

The 2,100 workers on strike in Asbestos would not allow the threat of homelessness to defeat them. On the evening of April 20, a group of strikers went to the neighbouring community of Stoke, where several strikebreakers lived. Once there, they cut the community's telephone wires and assaulted strikebreaker Gaston Malenfant. The men then invaded the homes of other strikebreakers, causing commotion, breaking windows, and beating occupants.[64]

"Such Explosive Possibilities": April to May 1949

The following day the population of Asbestos threw insults and rocks at strikebreakers on their way into the community. Barrette pressured JM to hold off evictions, but the local situation continued to deteriorate. JM president Lewis H. Brown responded by publishing a report on the strike (addressed to his company's stockholders) in every major newspaper in Canada and the United States, stressing his belief that the main issue in the conflict was union control over the Jeffrey Mine. There was no mention of health concerns. Blaming the CTCC rather than the workers, Brown wrote that the "crux of the strike is the insistence by the union leaders that they secure for themselves certain controls over managerial policy. It is the revolutionary doctrine that the right of owners hitherto unchallenged to select management to operate the property must be subjected to the veto power of union leadership."[65]

Since the 1937 strike, when workers succeeded in getting both P.P. Bartleman and C.H. Shoemaker removed from their positions and banished from the community, Jeffrey Mine employees had expressed their desire to have a say in how promotions were granted. JM had to some degree acquiesced by dismissing Bartleman and Shoemaker and establishing programs that would help local francophone workers attain managerial positions at the mine. The workers had yet to see any real progress on this front, and Brown's suggestion that the CTCC, not the strikers, was responsible for the demand angered the people of Asbestos. It was unusual for workers to have a say in company promotions, but according to the working-class majority in the community, that did not make it any less deserved.

Brown's report rallied the support of stockholders but did little to appease the people of Asbestos, who were still angry about the continued presence of strikebreakers and provincial police. Strikers continued their attacks on the houses of non-unionized JM employees; they also threw rocks through the windows of Mayor Goudreau's home.[66] Goudreau had disappointed the strikers by allowing the provincial police to remain in the community and by allowing strikebreakers to remain at the mine. Furthermore, the mayor was a member of the Union Nationale government, which was resolutely unsympathetic to the workers' cause.

In response to the strikers' attack on Goudreau's house, council voted unanimously to impose a curfew in Asbestos between the hours of 1 a.m. and 5 a.m. City hall would be locked each night at 12:30 a.m.[67] Police would arrest anyone found on the streets of the community past curfew, and the workers had to move their strike headquarters to the basement of St-Aimé. Council hoped this would prevent further violence in the town, but it did little to alleviate the growing frustration of the community.

Following council's resolution, more than five hundred wives of strikers went to St-Aimé to pray the rosary. This was hardly a radical act, yet the provincial police apprehended many of the women on their way out of the church and took them to the Hotel Iroquois, where they were interrogated about what Father Camirand had told them.[68] The women refused to give any information – if there was indeed any to give – and were released. JM clearly considered the priest a radical who was negatively influencing workers with socialist thoughts.

Townspeople were incensed when they heard that the police had harassed the women. Local union leaders went to council to demand that they control the provincial police, that they lift the curfew, and that they allow the union to pay for any damages the striking workers had caused.[69] The council agreed to consider this at its next meeting, but in response to the union's additional request that it forbid any outsider from entering the town to work at the Jeffrey Mine, it replied that it simply did not have the authority to do so. Council's inability to meet the union's demands led the strikers to believe that they would have to take control of the town by force.

The strike entered its thirteenth week at the start of May. Production numbers for February had fallen by almost half from 1948, from 48,873 to 26,148 tons. Anticipating how its stockholders would react to these numbers, JM claimed in the *Johns-Manville News Pictorial* that 750 Asbestos employees had returned to work. Aware that the magazine was sent to JM employees throughout Canada and the United States, the article's author also noted that if the strike continued, a number of factories would have to be closed and "as many as 100,000 employees will be thrown out of jobs, resulting in suffering and hardships not only to themselves but also to their families numbering perhaps 400,000 more."[70] By highlighting the broader impact of the strike and the potential victims beyond the boundaries of the town, the company was shifting the focus away from Asbestos. The article also emphasized how important the community was to the global success of the industry: while strikers did not want 400,000 people to suffer, the international reach of their labour gave them bargaining strength.

JM was skilled at rallying outside support for its side in the dispute, but so were the strikers. Archbishop of Montreal Joseph Charbonneau instructed every Catholic Church in the city to raise monetary donations for those on strike, and Archbishop of Quebec City Maurice Roy followed suit. The archbishops also provided valuable moral encouragement. Charbonneau asked the people of Montreal to think of the mothers of Asbestos, who were so worried about being unable feed their children, and stated that the Church had a duty to intervene whenever the working class was threatened.[71] Making the strike a Church issue rather than simply an industrial dispute helped generate widespread public support. Financial donations were sent to the families of Asbestos, but the community needed more than cash to stop the sharp increase in anxiety townspeople felt after JM announced that the seven hundred strikebreakers working at the Jeffrey Mine would not only keep their jobs when the conflict was over but also threaten the seniority of strikers when it came to promotions.[72]

Anticipating violence, town council demanded that JM re-employ those on strike when the conflict had ended and return them to their previous positions in occupation and rank so the local economy would not suffer more than it already had.[73] Council did not have the power to prevent strikebreakers from entering the town, but it could try to reason with JM in a way that angry workers could not. The threat to retain strikebreakers at the Jeffrey Mine implied that fully one-third of those on strike would be out of work when the dispute ended. The single-industry town could not support that great a number of unemployed men and women.

Council's request was as close as it had ever come to dictating how JM should run the Jeffrey Mine. It also reflected the tradition of cooperation and negotiation that company and community had established over the previous decades. But this effort was not good enough for those directly affected by the strike, who were struggling to feed their families. Pelletier wrote that the workers wondered whether they could replace JM management as easily as the company seemed to be able to replace them. Despite this stab at humour, the presence of the strikebreakers enraged those on strike.[74] Frantic with worry over losing their jobs and homes to outsiders, workers were compelled to assert their authority over territory in Asbestos.

At 5 a.m. on the rainy morning of May 5, about eight hundred of the Asbestos strikers began to barricade the roads leading into the community. Loading pickup trucks and station wagons with lumber and other heavy materials, and parking them across the width of the roads, they had blocked all the entrances to Asbestos and the Jeffrey Mine by 7 a.m., when the strikers were joined by a number of fellow union members from Thetford. Their goal was to prevent outside strikebreakers from entering the town and any local ones from entering JM property. Asbestos was closed.

Positioned at the entrance to the mill just before 8 a.m., Pelletier saw thirty provincial policemen armed with machine guns, revolvers, and grenade launchers approach a large group of men picketing outside the mine in defiance of the injunction placed against them. The community had become a battleground. Before any violence could occur, however, more than one hundred women arrived on the scene and said the rosary as they slowly walked in the rain between the angry strikers and the heavily armed police.[75]

The image of this group of women is haunting. It conveys the strong Catholicism of the people of Asbestos and the determination of local women to be part of the conflict. It also shows the belief among those on strike that although they were breaking the laws of Quebec, they were justified by the laws of God. Five minutes after the women proceeded down the road to pray with other groups of strikers, the police launched tear-gas bombs into the picketing crowd, allegedly hitting Rodolphe Hamel's twelve-year-old son Jacques in the face. The gas was effective in clearing the gates to the mine but did little to disperse the gathering crowds at the road barriers, where picketers beat any strikebreaker who ventured too close and turned over three cars before lighting them on fire. Danville soon filled with those who were unable to enter Asbestos,[76] which remained closed and firmly under the control of those on strike.

Strikers maintained the barricades for the entire day. The group of praying local women continued to walk the streets of Asbestos, bringing food to those guarding the town as other strikers smashed windows at the homes of local scabs. No JM official was harmed, but provincial policemen were. Targeting them as invaders of their community, strikers attacked and disarmed any policeman who came close to the barricades, overturned a patrol car, and broke the arm of Lieutenant Émile Contant as his vehicle drove away from the "wet, determined" strikers.[77] CTCC secretary Jean Marchand was not in Asbestos on 5 May, and the union had not sanctioned the barricades or the violence – like the call to strike, this was something that had come directly from Jeffrey Mine workers.

The policemen who had not retreated from the barricades were taken by the strikers and forced to march through the streets of Asbestos with their hands up until they arrived in the basement of St-Aimé. Police later reported to the *Globe and Mail* that the strikers led eight policemen to a platform in the church, where they were booed and ridiculed by a crowd of four hundred. According to Detective Quevillon, "they called us everything you can say ... All had clubs. The women especially screamed and

kept yelling 'Beat them, beat them!'" Detective Therrien claimed that
he was kicked in the stomach several times and that "you couldn't talk to
them. They just don't understand anything."[78] Father Camirand was
present, but told the policemen that the matter was between them and the
striking workers, not him. Camirand's willingness to witness these actions
without reproach, combined with the encouragement the women of
Asbestos gave strikers to inflict violence on the policemen, indicates how
strongly the local people resented the provincial police. It also shows how
violent the people of Asbestos had become during the strike. The strikers,
their families, and their priest believed that these actions were necessary
for victory.

Press helicopters circled overhead, and thirty-two media envoys waited
for more drama beyond the barricades, further adding to the war zone
atmosphere that had settled on the community. Few members of the press
were allowed into Asbestos that day; those already there were not allowed
out. Pelletier was a friend of the strikers, and so able to move throughout
the community; he had no intention of leaving. *Financial Post* reporter
Ron Williams, however, was terrified and tried to leave Asbestos. He got
past one barricade but was forced back by the second after he was pulled
from the car and told, "Too bad and I'm sorry, but if we know you, fine;
otherwise you stay."[79] Phoning the *Globe and Mail*, Williams described
the community as a beleaguered citadel under a reign of terror, and said
he was being guarded by provincial police armed with shotguns:

> There is a mass meeting going on in the basement of St. Aimé Church and
> everyone in the room is fearful that when it breaks up, violence will break
> out. As I speak, church bells are ringing. This is the first time in two months
> they have been heard ... I can see strikers patrolling the streets ... The streets,
> apart from the strikers' cars, are deserted ... I've never been in a situation
> before which has such explosive possibilities.[80]

Williams was terrified of what strikers would do next. Suddenly, church
bells were signs of danger and citizens on the street were supposedly violent
aggressors. Nevertheless, when the church bells stopped around 2:30 a.m.,
the meeting at St-Aimé dispersed and the strikers "vanished into thin air."[81]

The strikers had been "masters of the situation" throughout the day and
had intended to continue the barricades, but Camirand warned them not
to. He urged them to go home and rest, for it was futile to attempt to
defeat armed policemen and the next day would surely be difficult.[82] As
militant as Camirand's support for local workers was, his main concern

was for their safety, and he was wise to warn them. Hilaire Beauregard, the head of the provincial police, had requested more policemen from Sherbrooke and Montreal, stating that his force's patience had been exhausted in Asbestos. They would respond to violence with violence.[83]

The barricades were abandoned. The Thetford strikers who had come to Asbestos to help the community slept in the basement of St-Aimé while the local strikers went home. None of them were prepared when a contingent of 291 provincial police broke through the barriers to Asbestos at 3:00 a.m. Seeing only a few journalists wandering the streets, they decided to reclaim sections of the town. Their first target was St-Aimé.

The police arrived at the church at 4:00 a.m. as the men – almost forty of them – were waking. Led by Detective Daniel Nadeau, who had been injured by picketers the day before, they stormed the basement. A striker immediately struck Nadeau with a wooden club. Heavily outnumbered by the police, the waking men ran towards the stairs to the chapel, where they felt they would be safe. An officer hit Thetford worker Laurent Bernatchez from behind on the stairs and punched him until he lost consciousness. The press photographed him as police led him from the church. He asked the officers if he could go to the hospital, but they took him to the Hotel Iroquois instead.

The church, so important to the citizens of Asbestos, had been invaded. Pelletier reported that the police had been so violent that the church had been defiled by blood.[84] Shocking as this was, there was more to come. After police had rounded up the forty men, Justice of the Peace Hertel O'Bready read the Riot Act on the front steps of St-Aimé, forbidding anyone to gather in groups of more than two. O'Bready urged the small crowd before him to return to work. What occurred at the church would be described by the *Globe and Mail* as "an action without parallel in Canadian history."[85] If reporters were horrified by the actions of the provincial police, the people of Asbestos were terrified. Their place of worship had been defiled, and they were prisoners in their own homes.

Before the townspeople had time to react to the violence at the church, provincial policemen escorted strikebreakers into the community and through the gates of the Jeffrey Mine. Police then raided the homes of strikers and the local businesses where they had gathered, arresting 125 citizens and taking them to the Hotel Iroquois. The streets of Asbestos were deserted – in sharp contrast to the day before – as policemen patrolled them. The war zone atmosphere in Asbestos continued, but this time the invaders were in control. The local paper took the eerie calm as a sign that the strike was over, but this was far from the case.[86]

The treatment of arrested strikers by the provincial police was later revealed to have been ordered by JM officials who were present at the Hotel
Iroquois. Court records compiled in subsequent actions for brutality give
an account of what the strikers experienced. Police took Joseph Beaudoin,
Bruno Champagne, Alfred Blanchette, and other strikers eating in a local
restaurant to the Hotel Iroquois for questioning before they were sent to
jail in Sherbrooke or Montreal. Each man was taken to a washroom in the
boarding house and beaten into unconsciousness during interrogations
meant to find out who had put up the barricades. Beaudoin was fifty-five
years old and had worked for JM for twenty-seven years. During this
process, police also verbally berated these men and threatened them with
death. Worse than this, according to the resulting testimony, was the way
the police talked about Father Camirand.[87]

The police viewed Camirand as a dangerous influence in the community, although they could not attack him publicly. Both Willie Champagne
and Gérard Chamberland of Thetford claimed that police had insulted
the priest during the violence at the Hotel Iroquois.[88] The strikers emphasized this in their testimonies against the police because it supported the
idea that they were morally justified: the priest supported the workers
while company-paid provincial police defied the laws of the Church by
treating Camirand with disrespect. In 1949 Catholic Quebec, this was a
serious offence with the power to sway public opinion in favour of the
workers.

The police appeared to take pleasure in assaulting the strikers, but not
all of those under JM control agreed with what was happening. Several
men were allegedly beaten at JM's hospital in Asbestos rather than at the
Hotel Iroquois, including Jean-Noël Hamel, the son of local union leader
Rodolphe Hamel. These men were beaten severely and required stitches
on their limbs, torsos, and heads. Dr. Smith took X-rays to make sure their
skulls had not been fractured, gave them food, and confidentially told
them he was on the side of the strikers and disapproved of the way JM
was treating them.[89] While we cannot be sure Smith actually said this, his
efforts to convince JM to reduce the amount of dust at the Jeffrey Mine
suggest that he did sympathize, at least somewhat, with the workers even
as he published false medical reports on their supposed good health. It
also illustrates how Jeffrey Mine employees liked and trusted Smith, even
though LeDoux's report on asbestosis suggested that the company doctor
had been hiding the true state of their health from them.

Smith offered the injured strikers beds in the infirmary while he guarded
the door as they slept before being transported to Sherbrooke. Because of

this alleged support, Smith was the only JM employee not on strike who emerged from the conflict with a positive reputation in the community, and this impacted how townspeople viewed their health and safety at the Jeffrey Mine. Of course, the townspeople did not realize the extent to which Smith had helped JM cover up the damage the mineral was doing to their bodies.

The events in the Hotel Iroquois are indicative of how JM attempted to reassert its authority in Asbestos. C-JM president G.K. Foster supervised many of these interrogations and did not intervene to stop the violence.[90] The workers interpreted this inaction as approval, and Foster's presence revealed to them just how connected JM was to the police and to Duplessis.

Most of the local strikers beaten on 6 May were released on the condition that they downplay the bruises on their bodies, saying they were nothing but sunburns, that they leave Asbestos until the strike was over, and that they not attend Camirand's masses. The release of local strikers suggests that JM was reluctant to arrest them because it would go against the company's public statement that Thetford workers had erected the barricades, not those from Asbestos.[91] The families and friends of the men taken by the police had no idea what was happening to them at the Hotel Iroquois. The *Globe and Mail* described Asbestos that afternoon as a deserted city with blood-spattered streets. Pelletier reported that local women were frantic with worry about their husbands and sons.[92] Uncertainty reigned in the community, and Camirand spent the day going from home to home comforting families. No one knew how the police had used his name to justify their violence. In total, 150 men were sent from Asbestos to Sherbrooke; 53 were then sent on to a Montreal jail due to lack of space.

UNEASINESS AND BITTERNESS: MAY TO JUNE 1949

The events of 5 and 6 May changed Asbestos in ways that the first few months of the strike had not. *La Tribune* reported that "uneasiness and bitterness reigned" in the community, where the strike was entering its fourth month.[93] This sentiment contrasted sharply with the jovial spirits that strikers had shown at the start of the conflict. The town was on edge. The community-wide element of the strike was reinforced when the imprisoned men were released from the Hotel Iroquois and the Sherbrooke jail. These men were husbands, fathers, sons, and friends, and they remained in their homes for days to hide their injuries. Despite this, the community still saw their swollen faces, which generated strong anger and disgust throughout the town.[94] JM's image in Asbestos had been damaged throughout the strike, but it worsened as townspeople became aware of the violence that Foster had sanctioned at the Hotel Iroquois. The company had been an important presence in Asbestos since 1918; after these events, company-community relations would be far from harmonious.

JM continued to blame radical union leaders and Thetford miners for putting up the barricades in Asbestos. The Thetford workers were convenient scapegoats because they were not connected to the community in the same way Jeffrey Mine workers were. They were not friends or neighbours, and it was easier to blame strangers for the violence than it was to blame locals. Furthermore, it made sense from a public relations perspective to foster the idea that JM's workers were not violently against company policy and decisions.

Thetford workers had been present during the violence, but they had not raised the barricades. The JM workers had begun the strike on 13 February with clear goals in mind, and they had fought against the presence of the provincial police and strikebreakers in an attempt to gain control of the community. They had done these things of their own accord, often against the wishes and advice of their union leaders. Foster's attempt to take these actions away from local strikers illustrates how badly JM had understood its workforce.

On Sunday, May 8, 350 provincial policemen watched the people of Asbestos go to mass at St-Aimé. After mass, the crowd did not react when they were told the Riot Act had been lifted and that they were free to meet as they pleased. Camirand served as a spokesman for the people of Asbestos, and told the press that locals were appalled by the profane acts committed by the police in their church, which was now "battle-scarred as well as hallowed ground."[95] He also reported that the police had raided and eaten the donated food organized by Archbishops Charbonneau and Roy. Rodolphe Hamel had not seen his son Jean-Noël since he was taken on 6 May and did not know he was in a Montreal jail, awaiting charges with some sixty others. These men were unable to see their lawyer, Jean Drapeau, who sent letters of protest to Duplessis on their behalf.[96] A sense of the unknown settled on Asbestos.

The members of the press allowed into the community after the barricades had come down believed they knew what was to come: they waited with anticipation at the gates of the Jeffrey Mine on the morning of 9 May to see the strikers return to work. This did not happen.

The violence had not broken the strike, or the spirit of the workers. Hamel told the press that the workers were prepared to remain on strike for at least five more months. To ensure this was possible, the local union placed an ad in *Le Devoir* asking Montrealers to "adopt" a family in Asbestos by collectively donating $5 each week for every married couple in the community and $1 more for each child they had.[97] Hamel's confidence was remarkable, considering the violence that had occurred just days earlier and the suffering of the community after four months of strike.

The twenty-eight local men jailed in Sherbrooke were released on 9 May after the union paid their $800 fines. That night, strikers met in the basement of St-Aimé to discuss the brutality of the provincial police. Local union head Armand Larivée opened the meeting by highlighting the dedication of the strikers. After both he and Marchand spoke, Camirand told the crowd that their commitment to the strike was upholding the social doctrine of the Church and that their actions were ensuring that outsiders would not be able to steal their jobs. This removed any blame that could be placed on the strikers without denying their agency in the events of the conflict.

To combat this attitude, JM president Lewis H. Brown distributed a pamphlet on the strike to employees as well as to the press, which read in part: "It is our hope that every leader of every group in the Province of Quebec will read this report and from it obtain a clear understanding of the revolution that has been attempted by the leaders of the Asbestos Syndicate."[98] Brown had correctly assessed the main issues of the conflict, except that he gave agency to the CTCC, not Jeffrey Mine workers.

Brown wrote that the demands for workers to have a say in how land in Asbestos was used, how health issues were managed, and how promotions were awarded, were what the union wanted, not the Jeffrey Mine employees. He also stated that this was a conflict not over health or wages but over landownership. Quoting Pope Pius XI, he stated that "in the application of natural resources to human use the law of nature demands that right order should be observed. This order consists of this; that each thing has its proper owner."[99] JM owned the Jeffrey Mine and had the right to dictate how it was run, but the striking workers were the majority in this situation, and what happened at the mine directly impacted their health and their community. This, and the belief that the company depended on their labour for success, had instilled in them the revolutionary belief that they had the authority to decide how the Jeffrey Mine was developed. Brown did not understand this reasoning. The people of Asbestos should be grateful to JM. The company had spent over a million dollars on dust control equipment in the mills and another million on hospitals and recreation centres in the community. Brown could not understand that the

Jeffrey Mine workers could want more. In his mind, that was just not how single-industry working-class communities operated.

Brown blamed the violence of May 5 entirely on a group of outsiders who had terrorized the police and the people of Asbestos, especially the wives and children of JM officials, although no reports of officials or their families being targeted exist. His reasoning was ineffective in turning the opinion of Asbestos in the company's favour, if that was ever his intention. The squad of provincial policemen in the town numbered only fifty on the day the pamphlet was released. While this brought the population some relief, the knowledge that Foster and other officials had been present at the Hotel Iroquois while workers were being beaten weighed heavily on their minds. Pelletier reported that even those townspeople who had not fully sympathized with the strikers before the incident – specifically, local merchants and professionals whose lives had been caught up in the conflict – were now completely supportive of the workers.[100] Community dynamics in Asbestos continued to change.

For once, the local paper supported Pelletier's assessment of the town. While it still did not completely side with the strikers, L'Asbestos acknowledged the atmosphere of despair that had taken over the community. For its edition of May 13, the headline read, "Desolation Reigns in Asbestos." The story that followed stated that the first half of 1949 had brought a degree of suffering that the town had never experienced before.[101] There was no chance of alleviating this sadness, in the paper's opinion, because most of the population had not received wages for thirteen weeks, and in the meantime, JM had announced it would have to cut back its workforce owing to global economic conditions. This was a serious threat to the community, whose entire economy was based on the asbestos industry. The article concluded on a positive note, however, suggesting that the violence had ended the strike. Although workers were not yet returning to the Jeffrey Mine, many in Asbestos held this opinion.

CTCC officials did not believe that the workers were giving up hope and demanded a federal inquest into the role JM played in the violence of May 6. The union wrote that police interrogations had taken place in "torture chambers" owned by the company and had scarred some workers for life.[102] These claims were based on the testimonies of the arrested strikers, whose allegations against the police were believed by those who had seen their bruised faces. Jean-Noël Hamel, Gérard Chamberland, Alfred Blanchette, and Jean-Paul Houle, as well as some Thetford workers, were suing JM for $25,000 each for the abuse that had been inflicted on them. Adding to JM's worries that a public lawsuit would damage the company's finances and reputation was a confidential report given to W.H. Soutar, C-JM assistant mine manager, stating that cancer rates were rising in both Thetford and Asbestos, with twenty-two workers at the Jeffrey Mine having died of it between 1943 and 1947.[103] This concern was heightened in the middle of June when Dr. E.R.A. Merewether, the chief inspector of British factories, suggested a link between asbestos and cancer in an address he gave to the Canadian Medical Association.[104] Why Merewether did not transmit this information directly to Quebec's asbestos mining communities in crisis at this time is unclear, but JM officials were fortunate he did not. The company needed to resolve the strike in order to shift the press's attention off the industry before the threat of cancer was exposed.

Still unaware of the connection between the mineral and cancer, the people of Asbestos continued the pattern of life that had been in place since mid-February. Donations of food, money, and books continued to pour into the community but did little to alleviate local anxiety,[105] especially after strikers in the neighbouring community of St-Remi-de-Tingwick returned to work. While many took this to mean that all strikers in the asbestos region of Quebec would soon return to their mines and mills, JM was uncertain. In its June issue of the *Johns-Manville News Pictorial*, the company stated that the people who worked the Jeffrey Mine

> have lost more than $1 1/2 million in wages as a result of the strike. An increase in wages amounting to $5 a week would have been granted without any strike. With such an increase, it would take each employee over three years to get back what he has lost [but the] losses to the Company are much greater.[106]

The expense of the conflict had been great for the company, but few in Asbestos could believe that JM's suffering was greater than theirs.

The magazine also made it seem as though nothing was happening to bring an end to the strike. In fact, negotiations were constantly taking place even though workers had turned down a JM offer to raise their hourly wage by 10 cents on June 2. On June 19, the workers held a vote in St-Aimé on another proposed contract; 976 of them rejected it, and only 37 supported it. Pelletier explained that less than half the strikers had voted because many had been forced to take up employment outside Asbestos in order to feed their families.[107] The community had been shattered by the strike. The new faces of strikebreakers in Asbestos made this sad reality even more disturbing to the local population.

Adding to the community's worries was JM's announcement that it had discovered a new asbestos deposit near Munro, Ontario, and was moving equipment and $10,000,000 in development funds from Asbestos to this location.[108] This terrified even those who relied only indirectly on the Jeffrey Mine for their income. The entire community was connected to the mine, and even if JM's image had been damaged during the strike, townspeople needed it to survive.

Town council was hopeful that the conflict would soon end, but the strike and the Munro development soured relations between them and the company. No longer comfortable with relying so heavily on JM, council negotiated a deal with the Shawinigan Water and Power Co. to supply Asbestos with electricity.[109] Although this was an indirect way to articulate the new distance between council and company, it was clear that the community would function far differently after the strike than it had before the conflict.

Changes in Asbestos would also be great because of JM's demands at the negotiating table. Although JM claimed it had always treated its employees fairly, behind closed doors the company refused to rehire at least twenty of its striking workers who had been present at the barricades at the start of May. JM also insisted on its right to retain more than one hundred strikebreakers from outside Asbestos.[110] This would alter both the community and the spirit of camaraderie and authority the workers had at the Jeffrey Mine. When the Thetford strikers voted to return to work on June 24 after being offered a slightly improved contract, the people of Asbestos knew their strike would not last much longer; they were losing valuable allies and bargaining power for contract negotiations.

Their list of demands had been long in February; by the end of June, the strikers at Asbestos simply wanted JM to promise they would be able to return to work at the Jeffrey Mine. The issues the strike had raised remained, but the conflict had convinced the community that job security was the only thing that mattered. They could address the problems of health and land use in the future. The strike ended after 137 days, on June 30. An arbitration board began to negotiate the details of the new collective agreement – a risky but necessary move for the workers to make after suffering for almost five months without an income. *Le Devoir* reported that after the vote to accept the new contract at 1:30 a.m. in the basement of St-Aimé, workers and community members paraded and danced through the streets of Asbestos to celebrate the strike being over.[111] The morning of July 1 saw a continuance of the celebrations, with the church bells at St-Aimé ringing between 7:30 and 8 a.m. to summon a full-capacity crowd to Camirand's mass. Afterwards, Camirand expressed his hope that all community members – workers, professionals, and JM officials – would come together again for the sake of Asbestos,[112] which was optimistic considering how much the community had changed since February.

Townspeople were jubilant, but this was not the resolution for which the workers had sacrificed almost five months of salary and security. JM had promised to rehire all of its striking employees without discrimination, and they would be allowed to keep their seniority rights over the strikebreakers who remained at the Jeffrey Mine. In addition to this, the workers received what JM had offered at the start of April: a 10 cent wage increase, and four paid holidays a year, but no promises on dust elimination at the Jeffrey Mine, and no say in company promotions or in the technology used in the pit. The residual financial losses suffered by JM, the strikers, and the other businesses in the community would take years to overcome. The local newspaper illustrated the conflict between joy and sorrow when it announced the end of the labour dispute only in a small corner at the bottom of its front page.[113] Asbestos had undergone radical changes in land management, health awareness, and community power during the five months of the dispute, changes that would become increasingly visible in the months and years that followed the strike of 1949.

6

"Une ville qui se deplace," 1949–83

A s I stood on the observation platform overlooking the Jeffrey Mine on one of my first research trips to Asbestos, I was distracted from the pit by the sounds of children playing below me. On each side of the platform are piles of stone taken from the Jeffrey Mine, with asbestos still embedded in the rock. Two young boys had placed their bicycles against the chain-link fence that separates the mine from the town and were playing in these piles of asbestos, throwing the rocks up into the sky and taking much delight when they came back down and exploded in clouds of dust. When I drove away from Asbestos that day, foolishly holding my breath and trying not to rub my suddenly itchy eyes, the children remained, laughing and holding pieces of the mineral up to the sun, watching it sparkle and shine.

The town of Asbestos offers us an in-depth look at Quebec's second industrial revolution – one that focused on the technological transformation of the province's natural resource industries, not just its major cities. A major reason for the 1949 strike was that giant electric shovels had begun to replace workers at the Jeffrey Mine, which threatened the local inter-connectedness of people and land. These shovels took away not only jobs but also the traditional ways that a significant portion of the community had interacted with the land for generations.

In the years following the strike, the struggle over how land was to be used in Asbestos continued. This chapter examines the efforts made by the working-class majority of Asbestos residents to expand and maintain their connection to the land, the methods JM used to industrialize Asbestos

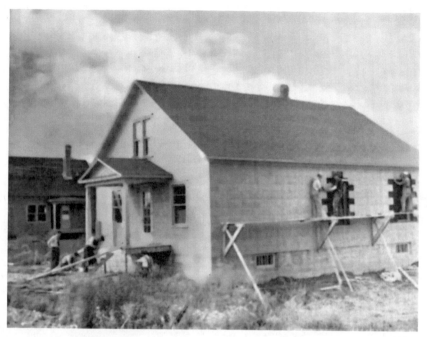

FIGURE 14 A family outside their new home, built by Chez Nous Ideal
Source: WG Clark Fonds, ETRC

and make it more "efficient," and the town council's attempts to mediate these opposing ambitions to ensure the continued development of the community. Land management in Asbestos from 1949 to 1983 was heavily influenced by fluctuations in the global market for the mineral, much as it had been before the strike. Now, however, townspeople resisted large-scale environmental change as the industry collapsed around them.

Following the 1949 strike, the people of Asbestos became increasingly focused on their authority over the land in the community. Central to this was a local commitment to become less reliant on JM for civic development and support, even though the local economy remained completely reliant on the Jeffrey Mine. Townspeople used the local Chez Nous Ideal, the cooperative home-building group they had formed during the Second World War, in new, more sophisticated ways to achieve this independence. Local residents bought shares in the group and pledged materials and five hours of labour towards the building of a new house for every member (see Figure 14).[1] These homes were independent of JM so that residents could control their own land and prevent pit expansion into the town if they did not believe it necessary. The strike had demonstrated the importance of homeownership when JM threatened to evict those living in company houses so that strikebreakers could inhabit them. Chez Nous Ideal became more active in Asbestos after 1949 and had a major impact on housing in the community, as well as on how town council made decisions regarding land use and development. The strike had driven home to the people of Asbestos the vulnerability associated with their dependence on JM.

STRUGGLE FOR OWNERSHIP, 1949–59

The strike had damaged the local economy, but it had actually been good for the industry, which was suddenly confronted with a shortage of approximately a quarter of a million tons of asbestos because of the Jeffrey Mine's months of inactivity.[2] The global demand and price for the mineral rose dramatically, and JM increased production at the Jeffrey Mine. At the same time, townspeople, JM, and town council purchased as much land as they could. Land in Asbestos had great value, and everyone wanted a piece of it. In the years following the strike, the land and the people who owned it constantly changed.

Town council anticipated the impact of the booming market on the community by annexing land from Shipton Township in August 1949 for a potential residential subdivision.[3] The council also purchased land from Shipton and individual property owners throughout 1949 so that it could expand the roads and boundaries of Asbestos, while pulling away from JM and the close working relationship the two had enjoyed prior to the strike. When JM asked council to repair the sewers close to the Jeffrey Mine in September 1949, the company was told that the issue would have to be put to a community referendum; before the strike, the council had agreed to almost everything JM requested. Also different was council's response to Chez Nous Ideal. When the home-building collective requested a reduced price on land to build twenty family homes and one thousand feet of new road and sewers, council purchased it from Shipton for them.[4] Then in 1950, community members demanded that the company reopen rue St-Georges near the Jeffrey Mine.[5] Prior to the strike, council had allowed road closures whenever JM requested them; indeed, it had relied on the company to modernize community roads by paving them. This was no longer the case.

An industrial boom in the 1950s returned to the community of Asbestos some of the confidence it had lost during the final weeks of the strike.

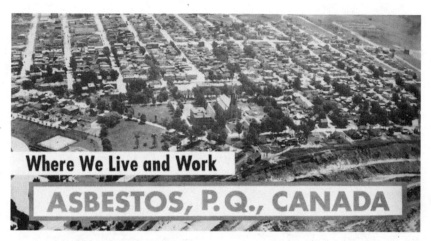

FIGURE 15   Featured photo of Asbestos in the *Johns-Manville News Pictorial*, 1950
Source: *Johns-Manville News Pictorial*, October 1950, 8, WG Clark Fonds, ETRC

Although the Soviet Union was emerging as a major source of asbestos, Canada continued to provide 61 percent of the world's supply, worth over $64 million.[6] Asbestos was not the only Quebec community mining the fibre, but the Jeffrey Mine deposit was by far the most productive, with workers extracting on average three times as much as those at Thetford.

The community's assertiveness challenged JM's ideas about how to manage single-industry towns. In many ways, the strike should have reminded townspeople of their reliance on the company. They were, of course, aware of this. Still, they drew confidence from the role they were playing in a global industry. Illustrating this, in October 1950 an article in JM's monthly employee magazine titled "Asbestos, PQ, Canada: Where We Live and Work" explained that because of the exponential production levels at the Jeffrey Mine and the seemingly infinite uses for the mineral, "asbestos serves nearly every man, woman and child at least once a day in our modern civilization (see Figure 15)."[7] As the leading producer of raw asbestos in the world, the Jeffrey Mine had global reach, and workers took great pride in this.

Despite workers' protests against the use of new electric shovels in 1948, JM soon introduced even more machinery to its Asbestos operations. In 1951 the company replaced the pit trains with giant thirty-five-ton trucks, which travelled continuously from the bottom of the mine to the top, loading and unloading fibre.[8] Even larger trucks were introduced as the years went on; by the 1970s, their capacity topped 200 tons. This new extraction technology continued to reduce the number of workers needed in the Jeffrey Mine. In addition to this, JM altered how shifts were run at the mine: from now on, "one shift of miners leaves for the washroom for a shower and change to street clothes before heading home as another shift waits to enter the cage" that would take them down into the pit.[9] The Jeffrey Mine had become an efficient, giant open-air factory: its workers were the tiny gears that kept it running, and the land was forever being remade in its thrall.

In the past, the people of Asbestos had seen the changes to the land at the Jeffrey Mine simply by walking by it, as the seemingly ever-growing pit was such a visible presence in the community. The block-caving system JM had introduced at the mine allowed increased production without more ground surface space. Each block was now two hundred square feet and had crushing plants 816 feet below ground, and loading facilities 950 feet down.[10] The company's latest industrialization of the land was both massive and subtle. It occurred throughout JM property but deep enough down that townspeople were not confronted by it as they had been by the open pit. This hid the march of extraction from most eyes.

By 1952, Canadian miners were extracting 1,000,000 tons of asbestos each year, fully 70 percent of the global supply.[11] The Jeffrey Mine remained the largest chrysotile mine in the world, and to process its output, JM spent $14,000,000 on the world's largest, most modern asbestos mill, fourteen storeys high and 75,000 square feet in size.[12] Jeffrey Mine workers were integral to these developments. Requiring only two hundred feet of new land for an entranceway, the mill was built on JM property and became an imposing presence in the community, visible from anywhere in town. By 1953, the global market price for asbestos was higher than for gold.

Throughout this industrialization of local land, Jeffrey Mine workers remained connected to the natural environment through their labour, and other community members remained connected to it through their everyday lives (see Figure 16). JM also possessed a close understanding of the land, however, and when town council and Chez Nous Ideal attempted to build one hundred homes on newly annexed land in 1953, company officials warned against it. JM had already considered building on the land, but it was an unstable mixture of sand and gravel, and there were several large, deep holes that the company had created while determining whether it had any value.[13] Council and Chez Nous Ideal suspended the project on this advice.

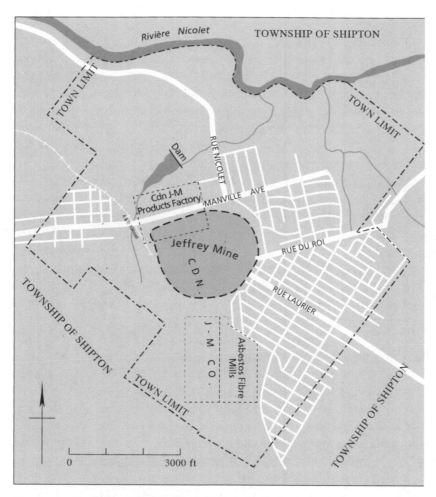

FIGURE 16 Insurance plan of the town of Asbestos, Quebec, 1953
Source: "Insurance Plan of the Town of Asbestos, Quebec, 1953," Collection numérique
de cartes et plans, ID# 174347_001, BANQ

JM demonstrated its expertise with land use both locally and globally.
Locally, JM dominated, preventing townspeople from becoming independent of it. Globally, JM prospered as the company that controlled
the Jeffrey Mine, 2,000 feet wide and 405 feet deep in 1954, from which
between 4,000 and 6,000 tons of asbestos were extracted each day.[14] Some
60 percent of the fibre that workers extracted from the Jeffrey Mine came
from underground caves, and JM's heavy investment in new technologies
continued to make the pit more factory-like. The giant trucks that hauled

the fibre out of the Jeffrey Mine along fifteen-foot-high spiralling benches made twenty-two trips to the surface during each of three daily shifts, five days a week, having been filled by massive shovels that required fewer men to operate.[15] JM also developed a new blasting method that used dynamite without wires so the Jeffrey Mine's fibre would remain pure (i.e., clear of foreign materials). These technologies replaced employees who for decades had blasted the fibre free with dynamite, gathered asbestos by hand at the bottom of the pit while picking out debris, and hauled bags full of raw mineral up the slopes of the mine.

JM's further industrialization of the land dramatically increased Quebec's asbestos production. By 1954, it had reached 914,864 tons, worth almost $80,000,000. These figures led the *Canadian Mining Journal* to state that technological advances would "ensure asbestos mining as a principal industry in Quebec for at least another century."[16] Wealth and stability came from the land at Asbestos. It seemed unfathomable that anything could impede continuing success.

Almost 10,000 people were living in Asbestos in 1955. Anticipating further population growth driven by the prosperity of the Jeffrey Mine, town council bought vast amounts of farmland for expansion.[17] Council paid for this expansion in part from the $900,000 in fees collected from construction permits, a portion of which came from JM as it built sixty-one company houses and seventy-eight garages.[18] Chez Nous Ideal was working towards local home ownership, but meanwhile, Johns-Manville continued to encourage its employees to rent more affordable housing from the company. This ensured that JM would have the power to move local residents when the company needed to expand the mine. JM also built seventy-foot-long tunnels that ran underneath neighbouring roads and buildings in order to transport the large trucks full of fibre without disrupting traffic.

Chez Nous Ideal remained active throughout the 1950s. It constructed 124 homes in 1956 alone, which made it, not JM, the largest provider of new housing in Asbestos. While home ownership was a sign of local prosperity, the longevity of these properties in the face of Jeffrey Mine expansion was questionable. If the *Canadian Mining Journal*'s prediction that the demand for asbestos would continue to soar for the next century proved correct, every home in Asbestos might be sacrificed to the Jeffrey Mine. The editor of the local paper, J.-O. Poirier, suggested that the pit might become so large that the people of Asbestos would have to live in the neighbouring town of Danville.[19]

JM was more concerned about profits than about community disruption or dissolution. Described by the *Canadian Mining Journal* as the "giant of the industry" because the Jeffrey Mine provided 60 percent of Canada's exported asbestos, JM reported record-breaking profits throughout the late 1950s.[20] Although the company had started to mine underground in the 1940s to minimize the expansion of the pit into the town, soaring profits and changed company-community dynamics led JM to focus development on opencast operations, which were more efficient and more easily industrialized than other forms of extraction. In January 1958, they presented the town council with plans for further lateral expansion of the mine into the town.

The expansion would be gradual but massive. Reverting to opencast mining meant that extraction would have to begin beyond the unseen underground "caves." Put another way, the pit's new perimeter would encompass a good portion of the "buffer land" between the mine and community that had already been exploited by tunnelling. In exchange, the company offered unused land farther from the pit, but this would fail to address the partial destruction of rue St-Aimé by the opencast expansion. This was one of the community's main roads as well as the location of the church that had been so important during the 1949 strike. Echoing its earlier reasoning, council agreed to the extension because JM was the main employer in the town and the development of the mine was necessary for the community.[21]

JM was explicit in its motives for expanding and did not pretend it would require new labour for it. Indeed, the company laid off eighty of its underground miners in July 1958 and forty more in April 1959.[22] JM also cautioned council against purchasing more land on which to accommodate a growing population.[23] Townspeople were worried. Lost jobs, annexations, and JM's increased reliance on new technologies at the Jeffrey Mine were clouding the future. Townspeople voted against a proposed annexation of more land from Shipton Township and awaited JM's next move.[24] It was quick and dramatic. The Jeffrey Mine moved into town, eating into rue Notre Dame and forcing the relocation of families and businesses there and from rue Bourbeau. Soon after, others living on rues Laurier, Panneton, Lafrance, St-Jacques, St-Dominique, St-Aimé, Legendre, St-George, and Amyot were forced from their homes as the mine perimeter swallowed up houses and excavations destroyed familiar scenes and memories.[25] JM financed new roads and housing to accommodate displaced families, and the new homes – a mixture of JM housing and privately owned – were much more modern than many of those they replaced. Even so, the disruption and the sense of powerlessness in the face of industrial expansion affected the lives of many community members.

"Asbestos Must Produce More Asbestos": 1960–71

By 1960, the Quebec asbestos industry was worth more than $100 million annually. JM workers cleared 12 million cubic yards of useless overburden from the land to extract 30,000 tons of fibre and 12,000 tons of waste each day from the Jeffrey Mine.[26] JM was conducting experiments to increase the durability of roads by adding asbestos to asphalt. Anticipating a further boom in the industry, the company added more shifts at the mine, to which the local paper responded, "Asbestos must produce more asbestos."[27] Soon, town council asked JM to pave the Asbestos-Danville Road with the new asphalt, and the Quebec government requested enough asbestos asphalt to pave all the roads and highways of the province. In 1961, the Quebec industry was worth over $130 million.[28]

Although they understood the imperative that drove mine expansion, the people of Asbestos quickly came to resent the destruction of the community's religious and commercial centres. Asbestos had already sacrificed the original core of the town, which included both a church and a commercial district, during the expansions of the 1930s (see Figure 17). Now home and business owners were refusing to sell their properties as they sought some resolution of competing demands for life and work space. Business owners on rue Bourbeau wanted assurances from JM that their profits would not be affected by the expansion. Other citizens worried that the growth of the mine would create massive amounts of "dead land." Facing an impasse, the company appealed to the Quebec government. Despite the provincial government's commitment to ending foreign control over the province's natural resources, Minister of Natural Resources René Lévesque forced the issue by declaring that he would pass a bill of expropriation mandating the expansion of the Jeffrey Mine.[29] Recognizing the inevitable in January 1964, *Le Citoyen* opined that unless JM was allowed to expand when and where it desired, the company would leave and Asbestos would become a "ville fantôme."[30] Townspeople had the choice between forsaking their homes and living in a ghost town.

Later that year the company paid the community $1.2 million for the church on St-Aimé[31] and provided land for two new churches, one of which would be named St-Aimé. The loss of the church was simply another chapter in the long history of physical destruction that had marked the twentieth century for the community. Townspeople seemed ready to give up their old church building and the bad memories of provincial police invading their place of worship in 1949, but the business owners on rue Bourbeau were less compliant.

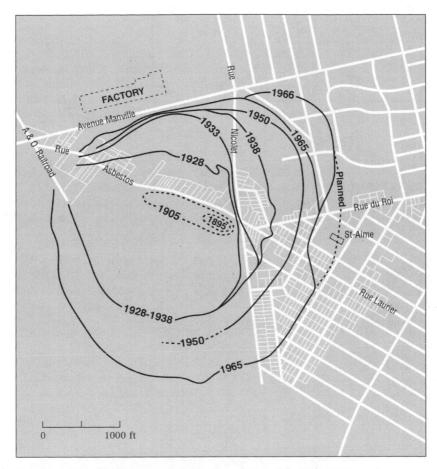

FIGURE 17   Showing the past and planned expansions of the Jeffrey Mine, 1967
Source: W. Gillies Ross, "Encroachment of the Jeffrey Mine on the Town of Asbestos,
Quebec," *Geographic Review* 57, 4 (1967): 529

The merchants of Asbestos did not want their businesses sacrificed to
the Jeffrey Mine. Many believed that the town would do better if the bill
of expropriation failed, and went to Quebec City to protest it. Their ap-
peals were considered, but the Quebec government was convinced of the
economic benefits of increased mineral extraction. Although the wider
region was beginning to see the town as the "dive" or "hovel" of Quebec[32]
because of its landscape, asbestos production was too important to the
provincial economy for the government to stand in the way of JM's plans
to expand the Jeffrey Mine (see Figure 18). In June 1964, the provincial
government passed Bill 195, Loi modifiant la Loi concernant la corporation

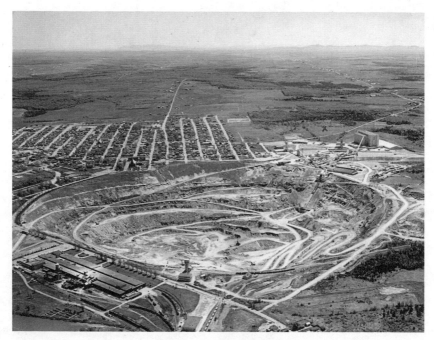

FIGURE 18 The Jeffrey Mine, 1965
Source: WG Clark Fonds, ETRC

du village d'Asbestos, authorizing the expropriation with the caveat that the company wait three years before expanding its operations in order to negotiate fair compensation with landowners – in particular, with the business owners on rue Bourbeau. Provincial politicians knew that the industry and the company were too valuable to the provincial economy to stymie, especially as the expansion project had an estimated worth of $20,000,000.[33]

While the government's decision was understandable, Asbestos residents who had acquired homes under Chez Nous Ideal refused to sell their properties to JM. In the end it was left to council to forcibly buy the land and sell it to the company.[34] The local paper urged people to think of the gains that would come from the expansion, not the losses. Asbestos had been founded on a tradition of building and rebuilding to accommodate the needs of the Jeffrey Mine, and because of this, it had become an exciting "town on the move."[35]

The global demand for asbestos doubled between 1955 and 1965, and the industry was worth over $148 million to the province. However, the people of Asbestos were growing increasingly disillusioned with JM's imperious actions. In April and May 1965, large rocks were hurled from the pit and into homes in the west end of town during blasting operations. The company claimed that it had invited the people living in at-risk areas to leave their homes when dynamite was being set off and that it was not JM's fault if they did not.[36] This was an effective, possibly unintentional way to get the people of Asbestos to sell their property to JM, but it changed how locals saw the Jeffrey Mine. For them, it was becoming an ever more dangerous and invasive presence.

By 1967, Asbestos was without a central district after the loss of 250 buildings to a surge of mine expansion that had swallowed 54 percent of downtown land.[37] Hearing of the exponential growth of the Jeffrey Mine, Gill Ross, a professor at nearby Bishop's University, visited the community and tracked the path the pit had taken into Asbestos, mapping it even as he attempted to grapple with the sheer magnitude of operations.[38]

Ross noted that while extraction levels had increased exponentially since 1949, technological advances had restricted workforce growth to two hundred. The town did not look on this favourably, but the *Canadian Mining Journal* favourably contrasted "The Free World's Largest Asbestos Producer" with the Soviet Union's growing asbestos industry. The journal marvelled at how JM had turned Asbestos into an "industrial complex" able to produce over 600,000 tons of the mineral annually.[39] The article praised the technological advances JM had introduced, attributing the industrialization of the pit to the rising cost of labour, the increasing size of haulage equipment, and the need to extract more rock because the quality of the mineral was decreasing.

Through all of this, the people of Asbestos maintained a strong sense of place attachment. During the 1967 St-Jean-Baptiste parade, local residents cheered a float proclaiming: "L'amiante notre patrimoine" (Asbestos: Our Heritage).[40] Residents objected confidently and strongly when business got in the way of community life, believing there could be a balance between the two. In April 1968, community members complained that they were being forced to "dine on dust and noise" by the expansion of the mine.[41] Citizens urged their councillors to reroute JM's expansion plans away from local neighbourhoods, or to establish a 1,000-foot buffer zone between the pit and the town. The new mining technology was louder, noisier, smokier, and more disruptive than previous extraction methods and was seriously impinging on the town's quality of life.[42]

Council established the thousand-foot buffer zone between the mine and the community in September 1968. This resulted in the demolition of more roads and houses, but also in JM giving $20,000 to town council for urban redevelopment.[43] In July 1969, a two-hundred-foot-long wall was constructed between boulevard St-Luc and the Jeffrey Mine. The wall marked a significant change in relations between the people and the pit. Once a place without a fence where children would play on weekends, the mine was now closed off from the community at the request of the people.

In September 1969, the Quebec government strengthened the towns-people's growing influence on the course of development by ruling that the relocation of boulevard St-Luc required by yet another phase of mine expansion could not proceed without local agreement.[44] The provincial government had finally recognized that the needs of the people of Asbestos were just as significant as those of the company. Although the town extended many roads away from the pit in 1970, anticipating further destruction of current neighbourhoods by mine expansion, this ruling encouraged JM to put mine expansion on hold as they deployed new technology to extract smaller, previously neglected asbestic fibre from the massive piles of pit tailings that had been part of the landscape since before the 1930s.

Because of massive mine expansion, housing was a major issue in Asbestos at the start of the 1970s. Although the town's population was not growing significantly, residents who were being forced to move because of the expanding Jeffrey Mine had nowhere to go. Chez Nous Ideal and the company had stopped purchasing new land and building houses. When JM told the Quebec government that the 1971 housing shortage was not the company's fault, however, town council lashed out, calling officials Pontius Pilates. Land use issues had once again altered community relations.[45] Many families lived in dangerous proximity to the Jeffrey Mine without any alternative place to go, but the company was refusing to accept responsibility for the situation. By now, officials were beginning to understand that because of the negative health effects of asbestos, the future of the community – and the industry – was limited.

The provincially run Société d'Habitation du Québec replaced the local Chez Nous Ideal and joined with town council in 1971 to construct 151 new houses in Asbestos. JM promised that these homes would be safe from the expanding Jeffrey Mine for at least fifty years.[46] That Chez Nous Ideal had given way to a government agency reflected the changed political landscape of Quebec. The new homes built by the society would be for families displaced or cut off from town by the growing pit.[47] The housing crisis highlighted the growing authority of the townspeople and the province when it came to deciding how to balance land and people in Asbestos. JM's role in the community was diminishing.

CHANGE IN COMMAND, CHANGE IN DIRECTION: 1972–83

As the 1970s progressed, signs of local confidence among the townspeople of Asbestos grew. One-third of fibre production at the Jeffrey Mine was now from pre-1930s tailings, but JM also wanted to increase the amount of asbestos its workers extracted from the pit. The industry was worth over $210 million in 1972, and the company wanted to raise yearly production from the mine to 700,000 tons by 1975.[48] This would likely have flooded the market with a mineral that the Western world was beginning to reject as awareness of its detrimental health effects increased. JM wanted to extract as much asbestos as it could from the mine before the industry collapsed.

The people of Asbestos vigorously opposed JM's expansion plans. The local newspaper termed the pit a "flawed mine" and reported the forced evacuations of citizens from their homes, which were falling into the pit.[49] Council soon closed sections of boulevard St-Luc for safety reasons, and JM announced that 160 local residents would have to move in order for the pit to incorporate part of the road. In response, the paper asked, "But where can they go?"[50] All 160 people refused to move. By now, the community was aware it would not be sharing in the profits that increased extraction would bring the company. Due to technological advances and a diminished global market, 154 workers were laid off in 1975.[51] In the 1930s, the townspeople had rallied behind the expansion of the Jeffrey Mine in the hope of getting out of economic depression; in the 1970s, JM's plans had a completely different feel and purpose. The industry continued to be worth millions of dollars, but as the world's opinion of asbestos changed, so did the importance of the Jeffrey Mine.

The company's rapid expansion of the pit and the refusal of families on boulevard St-Luc to leave their homes led to more accidents caused by rocks flying into the community during blasting. JM's rapid expansion plans also adversely affected the mine itself. In 1975, landslides destroyed large portions of the pit's southeast spiral benches. In response to the civic disturbance, town council demanded that the provincial government force JM to limit its expansion plans to protect the community.[52] The town of Asbestos grew increasingly dangerous as rocks flew through neighbourhoods at all hours. In 1976, projectiles from the Jeffrey Mine crashed into one of the few remaining stores on rue Bourbeau and struck the owner's son. Months later, a flying rock went through the roof of M. Hyppolyte's home on rue St-Barnabé and landed in his baby's empty bassinette.[53] The provincial government ordered JM to be more careful with blasting in the pit, but the company instead decided to invest $77 million in new equipment and a new factory that would further decrease JM's reliance on local manpower and increase its production levels by enabling more blasting each day.[54] Nothing would get in JM's way, especially the community, as the company frantically extracted as much fibre as it could while the industry was still viable.

Townspeople believed that the community and the mine needed to balance progress with stability. The town was not against progress, and it even purchased more land on which to expand in June 1977, but it was becoming increasingly frustrated with JM treating the people of Asbestos as though they were of little importance. In 1977, council described flying rocks as acts of vandalism and complained of rising gusts of dust that were so thick that life in Asbestos had become intolerable.[55] Flying rocks, thick clouds of toxic dust, and the constant noise of new machines had transformed the community into an industrial horror.

Yet, the company and its supporters were able to turn the damage the mine was doing to Asbestos into something positive. A 1977 *Canadian Mining Journal* article reported that over the next three years, JM would destroy more than two hundred buildings to accommodate the Jeffrey Mine's growth. The article excused these actions: "Asbestos is after all, a fairly old town and ... [This is] a form of forced urban renewal that has so far been to the benefit of Asbestos, turning it into a pretty well-planned town that boasts the latest and best in community facilities."[56]

By the mid-1970s, the Jeffrey Mine was well over a mile in diameter – 6,500 feet (or 2 kilometres) east to west, 6,000 feet north to south, and 1,000 feet deep. Its immense size made life in the community increasingly difficult. No longer caring much for community-company relations if they got in the way of production, JM continued to industrialize the land and the people who worked it.

By introducing the "hot shift change," the company ensured that the Jeffrey Mine would be worked constantly, with one shift ending only after the men starting the next shift had been dropped off at the bottom of the pit by a small truck, which would then deliver those done for the day to the top of the mine. This avoided the usual brief halt in production between crews.[57] JM also planned to introduce autonomous working crews, which would be stationed in mini-mines all around the pit. These crews worked together but had little contact with other Jeffrey Mine employees; many believed this seriously affected workplace camaraderie. Adding to the diminished camaraderie at the mine were continued layoffs, with sixty workers losing their jobs in 1977 despite JM recording the biggest profits in its history. Technological and organizational changes in the late 1970s had been great for business but bad for workers.

Layoffs and operational changes at the mine created a sense of unease in the community. This unease quickly turned to anger as the increased extraction rates enabled by the new technology made living in Asbestos even more hazardous than it already was. In January 1978, dynamiting at the Jeffrey Mine blasted three large rocks into the community. One crashed into the home of Adrien Sirois on rue St-Jacques; another, weighing twenty-three pounds, broke through the exterior wall of Yvette Boucher's house on rue Notre-Dame, 1,800 feet away from the pit; and the third destroyed the kitchen of another local resident.[58] Those affected reported JM to the police and the Quebec government. In their eyes, this was assault, not business or resource development. The province forced the company to establish set blasting times so that townspeople could evacuate their homes. Although not intentional, these accidents allowed the company to expropriate the homes closest to the Jeffrey Mine even though the owners did not want to sell. Marie Fortin-Drouin was informed in September 1979 that her house on boulevard St-Luc was no longer safe.[59] Although she obtained an injunction against the expropriation, town council forced Fortin-Drouin to vacate her home. JM employees helped her move. A week later, a rock blasted through the roof of the Desrochers funeral home and destroyed a ceramic figure of a praying Jesus. Cars and windows along boulevard St-Luc and rue Roi were also damaged.[60]

Such accidents angered the people of Asbestos, and they became increasingly resentful of the company. Townspeople maintained their rigid position against further expropriations and sought new ways to gain control over the land in Asbestos. In September 1980, council agreed to the relocation of boulevard St-Luc, rue St-Dominique, and rue Laurier, but told JM that the current plans could not be altered in any way, that officials would have to negotiate with every property owner individually for the sale of the land, and that the company would have to bear the cost of paving the newly relocated roads.[61]

Increased awareness of asbestos-related disease in the early 1980s hastened the collapse of the global market for the mineral,[62] and JM was losing its authority both locally and globally. In January 1981, frustrated with the constant noise and dust from the pit, a group of townspeople asked council if there was a municipal or provincial law setting a safe distance between residential buildings and the "cratère d'exploitation" that the mine had become.[63] Although this could have been a simple request for a new buffer zone between the pit and the community, the language used is telling. It was only in the early 1980s that the people of Asbestos started to look at the Jeffrey Mine as a crater: something that had happened to their land, not something they did to it. Local residents had always lived in close proximity to the Jeffrey Mine, but JM's introduction of new technology had decreased the interaction between workers and the pit, turning it into something mechanical and foreign. The people wanted to re-establish the local, historical balance between mine expansion and town expansion that this new technology had destroyed.

Despite local sentiments, the looming crisis in the global asbestos industry led the provincial government to support JM's industrial endeavours as long as they kept people employed. When council asked the province to establish a minimum buffer zone of 150 feet between the edges of the Jeffrey Mine and the community, the natural resources minister replied that doing so was unthinkable.[64] The 1,000-foot buffer zone the company had established in 1968 had disappeared by 1981, but keeping the industry afloat had become more important to the company and the province than maintaining the community. The economic strength of the industry was weakening, but the government continued to regard JM as a financial powerhouse. The province would not restrict development of the Jeffrey Mine. With the government's permission, JM continued to purchase individual plots of land throughout the community even while announcing that it would reduce its workforce from 2,200 to 1,500 in May 1981.[65]

Town council acknowledged the new reality of decline in June 1982, when it refused a plan for the Société d'Habitation du Québec to build ten new homes to accommodate citizens displaced by the Jeffrey Mine. Council justified its decision by pointing out that layoffs at the pit meant there would be an exodus of people from Asbestos to other communities that had both jobs and homes available.[66] People were leaving the community because the industry was collapsing. The community was extremely vulnerable to the international downturn of the industry, and many had given up.

Asbestos had suffered through economic collapse and depopulation in the past. William H. Jeffrey had declared bankruptcy in 1892. JM had closed the mine during the Great Depression. But the 1980s were different. Townspeople were not ignorant of the negative light in which the mineral the community was named for was now seen throughout the Western world; they knew the industry was suffering. Local fears were confirmed when JM filed for bankruptcy protection in the United States in August 1982. Since the early 1970s, Western markets had been shying away from asbestos because of widespread knowledge of its health risks, and the industry was no longer profitable. In response to the news of the company's bankruptcy, the local newspaper warned that without JM, Asbestos would collapse.[67]

Extraction levels at the Jeffrey Mine remained at 30,000 short tons of fibre each day, but many international buyers had stopped purchasing the mineral due to widespread reports of its negative health effects. Between 1981 and 1982, global sales of asbestos dropped by 26 percent.[68] Worried about the company's financial situation, town council demanded an immediate billing and payment system for land sales in 1983 so that the people of Asbestos would not lose their homes without compensation. It was time for the community to take control of its land and its future, both by insisting on immediate financial compensation and by participating in the creation of the Municipalité Régionale de Comté du Québec (MRC) de l'Or-Blanc, a new name for the region of the Eastern Townships of which Asbestos was a part.[69]

Renaming the region "white gold" at the height of the global rejection of asbestos was a defiant act that revealed Quebecers' willingness to stand behind the mineral. Townspeople balanced their memories of profitable glory days with their fears for the future as "it became very clear that the golden age of asbestos had ended and that a new battle has begun, more difficult still, for the survival of the community and its 100 year old industry."[70] In addition to this, "using its keen imagination to galvanize and revivify the community when it was in such great need, town council went out of its way, with surprising energy, to conserve what remained: its soul."[71] Council approved $45,000 to create the Musée Minéralogique in Asbestos in 1983. This featured samples of the fibre from the Jeffrey Mine in its raw, milled, and manufactured forms.[72]

JM left Asbestos at the end of 1983. It sold the Jeffrey Mine for $117 million to twelve former company officials who felt that they could manage the land, the community, and the industry even though the market demand for the mineral was continuing to collapse.[73] Townspeople's negative feelings towards JM's recent expansion of the Jeffrey Mine disappeared with the company's departure; residents of Asbestos declared 1984 the "year of asbestos." According to the town council, the community needed to revive the reputation of the mineral on which it depended for survival in order to redress the harmful effects of, for example, the US Environmental Protection Agency's campaign against asbestos.[74]

In a federal–provincial study on Canadian mining towns in decline during the 1980s, researchers concluded that locals developed an emotional attachment to their community. With this attachment "comes a sense of spirit and purpose, and commitment to a place ... Major layoffs or a closure may have a more severe impact than where such spirit is lacking. Another psychological factor is the uncertainty of being dependent on one major employer, and the probable lack of alternatives for employment in the immediate vicinity."[75] The people of Asbestos dealt with the terminal decline of their industry in ways that showed how deeply they were attached to the mine. Although money was certainly a factor, this was more than a simple desire for a paycheque: there was a deep sense of home and tradition rooted in the community, which connected townspeople to the Jeffrey Mine through the work they did and the lives they had led for over a hundred years. The future of the mine was uncertain in 1983, but community members were committed to its survival, even at the expense of their own health.

7
Useful Tools, 1949–83

IN APRIL 1997, FOUR men from Asbestos ran the Paris Marathon. Wearing T-shirts that read, "We Are Living as Winners," Michel Champagne, Guy Guerette, Pierre Laliberté, and Eudore Lemay sought to show the world that asbestos was not dangerous. France had voted to ban the fibre, and the runners had risen to the political challenge. Champagne stated that "my house is 800 metres from the mine and I am in great shape ... We want to prove to France that we live [in Asbestos] and are not affected by disease."[1] Like others before them, these men were attempting to use their bodies to combat overwhelming medical evidence that asbestos was dangerous. Their message was simple: if people from Asbestos could run a marathon, the mineral – and the industry – must be safe. When the men held a press conference at the Eiffel Tower, however, only four journalists showed up: three from Quebec and one from a French scientific journal. International opinion remained unmoved. But back in Canada, Prime Minister Jean Chrétien applauded their efforts. He also responded positively when busloads of residents from Asbestos and Thetford Mines arrived in Ottawa in September 2003 to demand continuing financial and public support for the industry. Government support was unwavering, at least until 2012, even though rates of mesothelioma – a particularly deadly asbestos-caused cancer – had increased significantly in Quebec since 1982.[2]

Mining communities learn to live with risk and danger.[3] JM buttressed this tendency in Asbestos by having company-paid medical doctors calm fears of disease. R.H. Stevenson and Kenneth Smith had assured Jeffrey Mine workers that they were healthy during annual medical checkups and union-supervised contract negotiations. Appealing to the benevolence of its workers, the company also promoted the idea that the mineral was synonymous with safety and that the community was helping protect the world from the dangers of fire. JM also sent the medical reports it had approved for public distribution – those that showed Jeffrey Mine workers were healthy – to the provincial and federal governments, strategically building its defence against a problem yet to be publicly identified.[4] When JM began to pull away from the health debate because of overwhelming evidence that asbestos was dangerous, Jeffrey Mine workers adopted the methods they had learned from the company to show they were healthy.

"Another Storm Is Brewing in Quebec": 1949–55

A major impetus for the Asbestos strike of 1949 had been increasing knowledge of what asbestos does to the human body. Having read Burton LeDoux's frightening exposé of asbestosis, workers knew better than to trust JM doctors, who had been instructed by the company to deny occurrences of disease in local workers. The strike had also sensitized JM's wholesale customers to the hazards of asbestos. Even as it was ending, JM vice-president Vandiver Brown heard from leaders of the Gatke Corporation (which manufactured asbestos-containing insulation) that "unless [asbestos producers] do something about [the health effects of asbestos] these little cases will breed like rabbits and they may grow as big as hares."[5] In agreeing to end the strike and return to work without any clear improvements to dust elimination at the Jeffrey Mine, the workers were conceding much to the company: they were accepting a risk that remains with the community today.

Committed to the position that asbestos dust caused no serious diseases, the company asked Dr Kenneth Smith about the health of Asbestos workers. Smith reported that 89 percent of the 708 employees whose X-rays he had studied in 1949 had been in dusty areas for more than twenty years and that only four of them had "normal" lungs. Of the remainder, 468 exhibited the early stages of asbestosis and 7 had full-blown cases.[6] These were shockingly high numbers, especially during contract negotiations to settle a labour dispute in which health issues were a central concern. But they were never shared with the union heads negotiating the new collective agreement.

In Smith's view, keeping the information under wraps was both sensible and humane:

> As long as the man is not disabled it is felt that he should not be told of his condition so that he can live and work in peace and the Company can benefit by his many years of experience. Should the man be told of his condition today there is a very definite possibility that he would become mentally and physically ill, simply through the knowledge that he has asbestosis.[7]

Smith seriously underestimated what the people of Asbestos knew about their own bodies. He further suggested that employees be transferred to less dusty areas of the Jeffrey Mine when their X-rays became alarming and "before there is any possibility of a claim for compensation being submitted and accepted."[8] But there were so many cases of asbestosis at the mine that not everyone could be transferred. Those who were transferred were not told they were sick and probably accepted their relocation as a matter of course, although it is likely that some linked a sudden job change with their decreased ability to breathe, especially in the wake of LeDoux's exposé. Even as he ordered employee transfers, Smith urged the company to invest more money in better dust control technology; he had noticed significant exposure in the community downwind of the mine and mill, and he feared that the entire town of Asbestos was at risk.

JM officials absorbed Smith's report with their usual combination of worry for their financial future and confidence in their ability to contain the situation. Company executive J.P. Woodard warned another JM official that "dust is causing significant lung changes in many cases, it largely being a matter of time" before serious health effects occurred.[9] C.M. McGaw, an official at the Jeffrey Mine, was significantly more concerned than Woodard. In the middle of contract negotiations, he forwarded Smith's unedited report to JM's head office, stating that it "shows our tremendous potential liability on exposure. Hope you can help speed approval of the dust control appropriation."[10] Although JM president Lewis H. Brown had claimed during the strike that the $1 million the company had already spent on dust elimination technology at the mine was sufficient, Smith's study frightened JM into approving an additional $5.5 million for better dust control. Woodard wrote to McGaw that he hoped "this will make a real improvement in your working condition situation, both within and without the plant."[11] Dust had become a community-wide issue because of the strike. Health reforms needed to be visible both at the Jeffrey Mine and throughout the town of Asbestos.

Despite Woodard's belief that the new funds for dust control would help ease tension in the community, JM kept both Smith's findings and the plan for improved dust elimination technology secret during contract negotiations. Admitting there was a dust problem would have proved that the company knew the mineral adversely affected its workers. Union heads would have used this to their fullest advantage. The company's reputation had suffered during the strike and would only worsen if townspeople discovered they were getting sick due to clouds of deadly dust. JM relied on the testimony of Dr. Arthur J. Vorwald during contract negotiations to dismiss local health concerns. Vorwald had acted as an assistant in the investigation of the lungs taken from dead Jeffrey Mine workers at the Saranac Laboratory in the 1940s, and he had taken over the directorship of the lab after Leroy Gardner died.

In the arbitration meetings of 1949, Vorwald significantly downplayed the severity of asbestosis. He testified: "I would like to compare lungs with our two arms, two legs and our two eyes. When one goes bad we can use the other one, and we have two lungs in case of disease."[12] When pressed by union lawyers who suggested that this logic meant that if a man without an arm was impaired, a man with asbestosis was as well, Vorwald replied, "No, I don't think so. He has an impairment of his lung tissue but he is not suffering from it." Vorwald's nonchalant attitude is especially shocking considering he had just instructed Smith to commission a confidential inquiry into the link between asbestos and cancer because cancerous tissue had been found in the lungs from Asbestos at Saranac.[13] Vorwald's testimony helped convince the arbitration board to rule in favour of JM. Better dust control measures were not made part of the new collective agreement in 1949, although the company did implement its $5.5 million investment in new technologies to control dust at the Jeffrey Mine in the months that followed. Limiting employee exposure to dust was becoming a priority for the company, but it did not want to acknowledge the risks workers faced each day at the mine in official documents, where their policy was to deny the health hazards at all costs.

Health issues took up ten of the fifty-seven pages of the arbitration ruling, far more than any other single issue. The arbitration board forced JM to admit that asbestos was harmful, but the company had full control over how it dealt with this fact at the Jeffrey Mine and in the community of Asbestos.[14] There was some debate over how long a worker had to be exposed to asbestos dust before he or she began to show signs of disease, and negotiators were uncertain of how much dust was too much. Neither the company nor the union leaders were inclined to think asbestos could be mined or processed without dust. Total elimination was never seen as an option, which reflected the community's acceptance of risk, and perhaps also a widespread, long-standing societal belief that mining was simply a dirty business.

When it came to the issue of asbestosis, JM medical professionals convinced the arbitration board that Smith's policy of removing workers from dusty areas when their X-rays showed signs of fibrosis was effective in stopping the progression of disease. They also claimed that these transfers allowed employees' bodies time to heal themselves. JM was confident that it could contain the problem at the mine and mill. Preparing a defence against another health threat caused by asbestos – cancer – proved more vexing.

Although Smith had not seen evidence of asbestos-related cancer in Jeffrey Mine employees by 1949, he was worried about the increasing number of international medical reports on the topic.[15] Smith restudied all the X-rays he had on file in Asbestos and told Karl V. Lindell, the new president of C-JM, that "if we are to defend ourselves in the compensation courts we must have proof."[16] Reflecting a marked case of loyalties divided between his employer on the one hand and his patients and the law on the other, Smith also instructed Lindell to ignore Quebec's new health regulation requiring occupational diseases to be reported, pointing out that the industry would be "unjustly penalized."

It was crucial that Jeffrey Mine employees were healthy. The town was the main source of the world's supply of the mineral, and JM maintained that the fibre was in its purest form there, as little processing was done at the manufacturing plant. When studies of workers in other locations found a link between asbestos and disease, JM claimed that materials or chemicals added after the asbestos left the Jeffrey Mine were the cause – thus placing the problem with the processor, not the fibre. This was a clever defence because manufacturers, especially in Great Britain, where many of the damning medical reports originated, usually mixed Canadian chrysotile with African crocidolite asbestos. So long as Smith could show that workers in Asbestos were healthy, the company and the industry would be as well.

The private correspondence of JM officials reveals that they were far from convinced by their own argument. At the beginning of 1950, Canadian lobby groups were pushing to have lung cancer recognized as an industrial disease, and Dr. Paul Cartier at Thetford Mines confidentially reported to Vorwald nine cases of lung cancer in his patients.[17] Smith acknowledged the potential threat of cancer when he told Woodard in

February 1950 that the lack of evidence of the disease in Jeffrey Mine employees did not mean it was not there. Woodard urged Smith to report on what his X-rays showed, so long as he was "sure" it would be favourable to the industry.[18] This was followed by a letter from Vorwald encouraging Smith to release his Jeffrey Mine data as a defence against damning medical reports because "another storm is brewing in Quebec, this time concerning a case of asbestosis with cancer."[19] Vorwald did not expand on who or where this case referred to, but he did not need to: the presence of asbestos-related cancer in humans, rather than in Gardner's lab mice, was worrisome enough.

JM had narrowly escaped catastrophe over the issue of asbestosis in 1949.Much like the tobacco industry at this time, the company wanted to avoid any suggestion that its product was carcinogenic.[20] Companies were not alone in this endeavour, and government officials had their own interests to defend. Asbestos was one of the most profitable industries in Quebec, and Premier Maurice Duplessis wanted to keep it that way. In May 1950, he eased JM's fears with an assurance that asbestos-related disease was not something with which his government was concerned. Duplessis publicly stated that companies had done everything humanly possible to eliminate dust in the province's mining communities, and that because of this, asbestosis was nonexistent in Quebec.[21] The government also took asbestosis off the list of industrial diseases for which the province would pay compensation.

The claim that asbestos was not only safe but helped ensure the safety of others was a common mantra during the 1950s. An extreme example of this came at the beginning of the decade when asbestos paste was used in heart surgeries to promote new, healthy tissue and blood channels.[22] JM was neither content nor complacent with this advantage, however. In July 1950, the company considered shipping raw asbestos from the Jeffrey Mine in paper rather than burlap bags to prevent dust from escaping during transport.[23] C-JM president G.K. Foster also met with QAMA, the lobby group formed by the province's asbestos companies, to urge them to fund a study on the link between the mineral and cancer. Foster was confident that by indirectly funding any study of Jeffrey Mine workers, the company would remain in control of the information discovered and released. In a letter to Woodard outlining company attitudes on these matters, Vandiver Brown explained that

we, of course, have never intended to suppress information obtained as a result of experiments financed by us, and on the occasions when we insisted that there be no publication without our advance "approval," we have had in mind that we might possibly wish to defer release until we could make such defensive moves as might be appropriate and available to us.[24]

Brown failed to mention that if a study was particularly damning, the company could defer its release date indefinitely.

JM deferred the release of the results of medical studies throughout its time in Asbestos. The company did so again when Smith notified JM of a new test for asbestosis developed by a Dr. Wright, who had visited the Jeffrey Mine in 1950. By measuring oxygen absorption in the blood of JM employees, Wright had been able to determine the level of pulmonary fibrosis in workers without relying on X-rays. Smith recommended that the company defer the release of Wright's study because it "might change our whole examination program and seriously affect the field of compensation."[25] Wright had claimed to have found at least eight definite cases of asbestosis in men to whom Smith had previously given a clean bill of health. The assessments by both Wright and Smith rested to some degree on human judgment. Wright established "normal" levels of oxygen in human blood as the basis for his calculations. Smith interpreted the shading on X-ray films. But before Wright developed his breakthrough method, Smith was the ultimate authority on the health of the workers at the Jeffrey Mine because only he had access to the X-ray data. Now it seemed that a simple blood test might destroy his reputation and authority in Asbestos.

The company also kept secret the report written by the former director of Saranac Laboratory, Leroy Gardner, who had emphasized the serious hazard of asbestos for human health during his study of Jeffrey Mine workers' lungs. Smith wholeheartedly agreed with this policy, especially after he discovered a case of asbestos-related skin cancer on Margaret Wolfe, an employee in the Jeffrey Mine's Textile Department.[26] The presence of cancer showed how serious the threat of dust was at both the mine and the mill. The company did not inform Wolfe of her illness, and in 1951 JM erased all references to asbestos and cancer from its Industrial Hygiene Meeting Minutes.[27]

Although job transfers and visiting doctors were not signs of a healthy workforce, Jeffrey Mine workers did not want another strike. They confronted the risks they suspected by continuing to work the Jeffrey Mine and by relying more on the opinion of JM doctors than on their own bodily knowledge. Even in the years following LeDoux's exposé, community members continued to trust the company's medical authority in Asbestos. JM had brought the town its first X-ray machines in the 1920s and had funded a new hospital in 1948. Examinations were running three to four years behind schedule because of the thoroughness with which company doctors now studied workers' bodies.[28] Without any knowledge of the degree of risk they were exposed to each day, workers put their trust in the company.

JM used this trust to its fullest advantage. In 1952, Illinois ruled that all asbestos products entering the state must carry a warning label reading: "'CAUTION – ASBESTOS FIBER' Inhalation of asbestos fibre over long periods may be harmful. The material should be so used as not to create dust or, if this is not possible, employees should be equipped with adequate protective devices."[29] Jeffrey Mine officials refused to put the warning on their shipping bags. What people did not know about the dangers of asbestos was security for the company and the community.

The 1952 interim report of QAMA's study on asbestos and cancer indicated that mice exposed to high quantities of asbestos dust quickly developed tumours.[30] In order to launch a pre-emptive attack on any non-industry-sponsored studies that showed the same thing, JM called on Dr. Anthony J. Lanza, Director of the Institute for Industrial Hygiene at New York University Medical Centre. While Lanza privately told company officials that Canada, not England, had had the first cases of asbestos-related disease fifty years before,[31] he publicly stated that the cancer and asbestosis rates being reported by E.R.A. Merewether in Britain were strikingly higher than those in North America. In Lanza's public opinion, neither of these diseases was particularly problematic when only Canadian chrysotile asbestos was used.

In response to Lanza's claims, Britain's leading asbestos producers, Turner and Newall, gained permission from QAMA for Dr. John Knox to visit Asbestos and Thetford Mines in 1952. In Asbestos, Knox found that there "has been a serious attempt to improve conditions in the mill here ... but as it is made to deal with more material than originally designed for, it is practically ineffective on that account."[32] Because of the large asbestos manufacturing industry in Britain, Knox was aware of the most modern methods used to prevent workers from being exposed to dust, which included a limit on the amount of fibre processed each day and a sophisticated wetting and ventilation system that prevented dry particles from floating in the air. Asbestos workers processed far more fibre per capita than their British counterparts, and JM operations could not possibly accommodate these new methods.

Knox found that safety standards in Asbestos were appallingly low, and he was unable to take a dust count measurement because the mill was too dusty for his equipment to work. He reported to Turner and Newall that the "weaving [department] was to me really shocking ... Good dust counting would have revealed a disturbing state here. There was no wetting ... and no exhaust used."[33] Despite the alarming state of the area where a number of local women worked, the company claimed that it had legal and medical evidence to disprove Knox's comments, and made no major changes in mill operations. Since 1918, only 8 percent of the Jeffrey Mine's total workforce had ever filed claims for occupational disease compensation. This was considered to be an insignificant number compared to what medical studies highlighting the dangers of the mineral suggested it could be.[34] For JM officials, this meant that asbestos had not affected the health of 92 percent of its employees. Rather than consider the possibility of severe underreporting of health problems in Asbestos, or the lack of compensation legislation in the province, JM used these statistics to bolster the argument that Canadian chrysotile from the Jeffrey Mine was inert.

Still, Knox's appraisal of operations at the Jeffrey Mine had some effect. Because dust levels could not be further reduced without great expense to the company, officials renewed their efforts to get employees to wear respirators. Since at least the 1930s, medical literature had recognized – and encouraged – the use of protective devices and dust control technology to reduce the risk of disease. On the ground in Asbestos, however, many workers refused to wear respirators because they clogged easily and restricted breathing. Employees also refused to wear respirators that were reused from shift to shift, and when personal devices were introduced, the company found that managers had to watch workers at all times to ensure they were being worn.[35] Although they did not know about the threat of cancer, it is telling that Jeffrey Mine employees continued to refuse to wear respirators even after LeDoux's exposé had made them aware of the risk of asbestosis. Workers did not want to get sick, but in order to be able to go to the Jeffrey Mine each day, they had to believe that asbestos would not harm them.

JM officials were puzzled that workers were refusing safety measures only a few years after a lengthy strike fought in part over this very issue. They were also worried about the long-term health and financial effects of workers not wearing respirators. Promoting a healthy workforce was especially important to asbestos companies in 1955 because new international medical reports were directly linking asbestosis and lung cancer.[36] Dr. Richard Doll, a contemporary of Knox's, had conducted an epidemiological study of British factory workers in Turner and Newall's operations and found direct links between asbestos and cancer. He concluded that male asbestos workers who had been in the industry for twenty or more years had a ten times greater risk of developing lung cancer than the general public.[37] This was a damning assessment, and in the original report he submitted to the *British Journal of Industrial Medicine*, Doll doubted that the risk asbestos posed to workers had been eliminated by improved factory conditions.[38] When Turner and Newall refused consent for publication of this conclusion, Doll changed the final sentence to read: "The risk has become progressively less as the duration of employment under the old dusty conditions has decreased."[39] This was a subtle yet significant change, one that continued the industry's trend of manipulating both medical professionals and the evidence they produced.

JM did this as well. Kenneth Smith's 1949 assessment of the health of Jeffrey Mine workers was published in 1955, after thorough editing by the company. Smith's original report had stated that only four workers had "normal" X-rays, yet the published piece claimed that 91 percent of the men he studied had no signs of asbestosis.[40] It went on to state that of the fifty-two employees who showed signs of pulmonary fibrosis, none had signs of asbestosis and many of them had worked at the Jeffrey Mine for twenty to forty years. Smith had identified the seven worst cases in his sample as sufferers from "full-blown" asbestosis, yet the published report suggested that only seven employees had it, and that none of them were impaired in any way. According to the published report, few employees exposed to chrysotile asbestos developed any signs of fibrosis, and those that did have asbestosis "have been known to carry on their usual work and live fairly comfortable lives for several years."[41]

"'Ignorance Is Bliss' Has Been Expensively Disproved": 1955–72

Smith's work was taken seriously within the Canadian medical community, which had difficulty making inroads in Quebec because of linguistic differences. His study convinced many Canadian doctors that asbestosis was a rare, non-fatal disease,[42] but JM continued to fret over the results of a QAMA study on the links between asbestos and cancer led by Drs. Daniel C. Braun and T. David Truan. Braun somehow tried to make the study's findings positive when he wrote to industry representative H.M. Jackson in 1957. He stated that of the ninety-nine cases of asbestosis and lung cancer studied, only nineteen of them were miners, which suggested that "the possibility of an association between lung cancer and asbestosis is much more likely to exist in asbestos factories than in mining operations."[43]

Industry leaders and public health workers could still see the Jeffrey Mine as safe, even if other medical professionals continued to show that asbestos was dangerous.

JM was not reassured by Braun's statement that milling asbestos was more dangerous than mining it. QAMA took this information out of the final "Braun-Truan Report" before its publication. In the confidential draft Braun and Truan submitted to JM in 1957, the researchers stated that they believed company doctors considerably underreported incidences of asbestosis and that this directly led to an increase in asbestos-related lung cancer.[44] There was no way JM would sanction the publication of this information. Braun and Truan concluded in their draft that independent medical professionals, not company-paid doctors, should evaluate the X-rays of all asbestos workers[45] – which suggested that company doctors were partly responsible for the increased occurrence in asbestos-related cancer because companies had instructed them not to report the first signs of illness. This serious accusation highlighted the very real problems of medical care in Asbestos. But the sanitized copy of this report released by JM in 1958 pointed to the smoking habits of miners rather than dust exposure or negligent medical professionals as the cause of such health problems.

Braun and Truan studied 2,273 workers in Asbestos who were alive in 1950. Most of them were under forty-four years old and smoked more than five cigarettes a day. Over the five years of the study, three of the forty-nine Asbestos workers who passed away died of lung cancer: "A.J." was a sixty-six-year-old smoker who had worked for twenty-six years in a moderately dusty environment; "N.O." was a sixty-five-year-old smoker who had spent thirty-four years in a mildly dusty area; and "R.M." was a sixty-five-year-old smoker who had worked thirty-seven years in the same mild section of the Jeffrey Mine as "N.O."[46] These numbers allowed the researchers to conclude that there was a higher probability of those with asbestosis getting cancer: "The mortality rate from lung cancer does not appear to increase with length of exposure or with degree of exposure, a fact which presents strong evidence against the carcinogenicity of asbestos. On the other hand, the study indicates that cigarette smoking is a very important factor in the incidence of cancer of the lung."[47] The study also stated that none of the 1,265 non-smokers at the Jeffrey Mine developed lung cancer.

Braun and Truan would have seen the unique type of lung cancer that asbestos causes, but they had been hired to boost the industry's image, not expose its risks. The tobacco industry, which had much in common with the asbestos industry, became a convenient scapegoat for asbestos companies looking to preserve the image of asbestos as safe. Both tobacco and asbestos were culturally embedded in Western society, and consumers associated both with modern, easy living. In the mid-twentieth century, medical researchers were increasingly forging links between both products and cancer, and asbestos companies saw this as an opportunity to diminish the growing evidence against the mineral. This strategy was intrinsically tied to negative societal stereotypes about the lifestyle choices of the working class. Of course miners got cancer: they smoked! Although Smith knew how hazardous asbestos was, he wrote that "this publication should form the basis for future surveys and reports" and would be a great tool to refute the studies of other medical professionals who did not have such a concentrated cohort of bodies to study.[48]

The *American Medical Association Archives of Industrial Health* accepted the Braun-Truan report for publication. Editor Herbert E. Stokinger wrote: "I, myself, was particularly pleased to learn the main conclusion of the paper was against the association of lung cancer with asbestos, for I had come to a similar conclusion on obviously far less information but was afraid to say so for this reason."[49] The bodies of the workers at the Jeffrey Mine remained useful tools for ensuring the legitimacy of the asbestos industry. Braun and Truan knew nothing of the post-retirement cases being secretly studied at Saranac Laboratories, where researchers had discovered over seventy cases of unreported lung cancer among Quebec's asbestos workers by 1958.[50]

This information is crucial to understanding how the people of Asbestos viewed their bodies. They knew they had respiratory problems because of their work at the Jeffrey Mine, and they had not forgotten LeDoux's 1949 exposé on the industry, but they did not know about the risk of cancer. The Braun-Truan Report bought the industry time and helped dull the impact of international medical studies that linked asbestos to cancer. Capitalizing on this, JM launched a series of print advertisements supporting the idea that asbestos was safe. One ad featured a baby sitting on a floor and saying, "What do you mean I'll catch cold on the floor? Our house is insulated with Johns-Manville Spintex!" The late 1950s also saw the launch of "Jim Asbestos," a JM mascot in a lifeguard uniform that instructed consumers on how the mineral helped make everyday products safer.[51] The message was clear: asbestos saved lives; it did not take them away.

These medical reports and advertisements worked to maintain the safe image of the mineral and the economic success of the industry. Despite the outward calm, however, JM was encountering difficulties in Asbestos.

In a letter to company headquarters, Jeffrey Mine executive J.R.M. Hutcheson wrote that "a possible health hazard is only part of the problem. We have the ever-present, and increasingly onerous problem of public and industrial relations. This facet of the problem is serious enough, the mere suggestion of a health hazard on top of the present problem would make the necessity that much more urgent."[52] Hutcheson's letter reveals that workers knew they were getting sick and that they did not believe JM was particularly concerned about their health. Company-community relations had not improved since the 1949 strike. Workers were willing to accept some risk, but it was not because of affection for the company.

By 1960, the link between asbestos and cancer was beginning to be better known among the general public.[53] Furthermore, medical studies on asbestos factory workers were beginning to show that lung cancer was only the start of what the mineral could do to the human body. For generations, the literature on the health effects of asbestos had centred on the respiratory system, but the 1960s brought a new challenge to company assertions that the mineral was safe. In an article published in *The Lancet* on December 3, 1960, E.E. Keal listed the deaths of men and women suffering from asbestosis in British processing and manufacturing plants over a long period. Most male subjects with asbestosis died of carcinoma of the lung, but most female asbestos-related deaths were caused by carcinoma of the ovary and breast, which suggested a unique interaction between asbestos and the female body.[54]

Joan Ross performed a confidential study on female workers at the Jeffrey Mine in 1944, after complaints about their high rate of absenteeism. Since then, none of the JM-sanctioned medical reports had mentioned the female employees in the dusty Textile Department at the mine, which Braun and Truan reported as one of the most dangerous places to work. Miners, medical researchers, and industry leaders had often assumed – perhaps even romanticized – that it was *male* workers who were at risk in such a masculine industry. Female workers were a different story altogether. Townspeople knew that female workers had significantly high absenteeism rates at the Jeffrey Mine; even so, they would likely have been horrified by the information in Keal's report. But a British medical journal was not something to which the Jeffrey Mine's francophone workforce had access. Furthermore, neither the English nor the French medical communities in Canada had published on the link between asbestos and cancer before 1965. Indeed, the mineral was only mentioned once between 1955 and 1965 in the *Canadian Medical Association Journal*, and then only in connection with asbestosis, not cancer. There were two mentions of mesothelioma, in

1957 and 1959, but researchers did not acknowledge the link between this cancer and the mineral responsible for it.[55] Asbestos and the Canadian public were isolated from Keal's discovery, and the company could manage local complaints without informing Jeffrey Mine workers of the health risks recently revealed by British research.

JM's main strategy was to insist that the pure asbestos taken from the Jeffrey Mine was not carcinogenic. At the same time, the company sponsored more medical studies of Jeffrey Mine workers. In a memo to managers about the compensation litigation suits that American workers were launching against the company, JM president C.B. Burnett wrote that simply saying "'no one has been hurt' is to ignore a basic management responsibility of getting the facts upon which to make a decision. The old adage 'ignorance is bliss' has been expensively disproved."[56] JM could not afford people knowing that Jeffrey Mine fibre was dangerous, but at the same time, officials were increasingly aware that denying the harmful effects of asbestos was a losing strategy. The company needed to know the complete progression of asbestos-related disease if it was to be prevented – which was the only thing that could keep the industry alive. The following year, Dr. Kenneth Smith, who had left Asbestos but continued to work for the company, went further than Burnett by asking whether JM was comfortable continuing "to impair the health of men and women [throughout its operations, and] to shorten their lives by our actions."[57]

Smith knew it was only a matter of time before the health effects of asbestos were exposed. Indeed, Dr. Irving J. Selikoff at Mount Sinai Hospital in New York was working on just such an exposé. In 1964, he published a report on 632 American asbestos insulation workers that concluded that steady exposure to asbestos led to increased rates of cancer of the lung, pleura, stomach, colon, and rectum. In other words, asbestos-related disease went beyond the respiratory system. His report also noted that the "incidence of more than 1 percent of deaths from pleural mesothelioma is strikingly high for a tumor which is generally considered to be extremely rare."[58] Mesothelioma is a fast-acting cancer of the lining of major organs, such as the lung, heart, and abdomen, and this study implied that asbestos was making it more common. Selikoff also directly refuted the conclusions Braun and Truan had made in 1957 when he wrote that "the smoking habits of the asbestos workers cannot account for the fact that their lung-cancer death rate was 6.8 times as high as that of white males in the general population."[59] His findings discredited JM and QAMA reports that claimed cigarettes, not asbestos, harmed workers, and his study received a lot of press because of it.

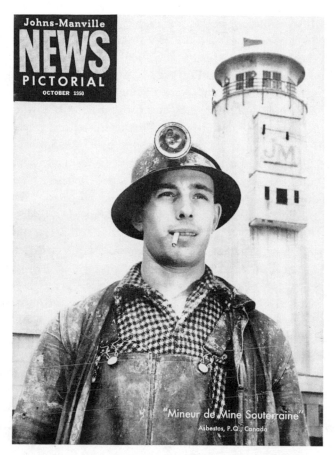

FIGURE 19   Cover of the *JM News Pictorial* depicting a Jeffrey
Mine worker, October 1950
Source: Johns-Manville News Pictorial, October 1950, WG Clark
Fonds, ETRC

This was a serious threat to JM's health propaganda campaign, which relied on the connection between cigarettes and cancer to maintain that the mineral was safe. The company had even used a picture of a smoking Jeffrey Mine worker on the cover of its newsletter to shareholders in 1950 (see Figure 19). Of all those connected to JM, however, Smith seemed to take Selikoff's study the worst. Condemning Selikoff as "ambitious and unscrupulous and ... out to make a name for himself at the expense of the asbestos industry," Smith reiterated that Jeffrey Mine employees were healthy and had none of the malignancies Selikoff claimed were common in asbestos workers. He then related how Selikoff acted when JM allowed him to visit Asbestos years before: "he told Dr. Grainger in a rather pompous manner that Grainger didn't know anything about reading [X-ray] films and that he, Selikoff, in that short period of time had seen much more disease than he imagined existed."[60] Again Smith was caught in a contradiction. He regretted that Jeffrey Mine workers were being put at risk, but he did not want his medical authority questioned any more than he wanted JM's reputation to be tainted by health-related revelations.

Selikoff's study of American factory workers challenged Smith's authority and suggested that the rate of disease in Asbestos was significantly higher than the company had reported. Smith claimed that the men Selikoff studied had been exposed to chemical additives and pleaded with JM to open the medical records of its employees to outside studies to prove Selikoff wrong.[61] Fearful of what other medical professionals could discover in these records, JM refused Smith's request. Despite this refusal, the company did acknowledge that the mineral posed some risk to human health when, in 1965, it began placing warning labels on shipments of asbestos insulation. These warning labels were not introduced in its Canadian operations, partly due to the absence of product liability law,[62] as well as the absence of worker agitation pushing for reforms. After the *Canadian Medical Association Journal* finally published an international study on the link between asbestos and cancer in 1965,[63] company official W. Hodgson wrote to JM's head office: "We have been assured by Dr. K.W. Smith that it is not necessary to use the caution label in Canada, and therefore, we obviously do not want it on any of our cartons."[64] Company officials considered placing stickers over the warnings on cartons of Superex pipe insulation sent to Canada, then decided it was too risky and chose instead to sand off the labels before they entered the country.[65] JM did not want to take the risk that its employees and other Canadians would see the warnings and turn against the mineral. The company needed Jeffrey Mine workers, as well as Canadians in general, to continue believing the mineral was inert in order to maintain production levels, industrial relations, and the false idea that Jeffrey Mine chrysotile was safe.

JM initiated a new QAMA study of Quebec asbestos workers in 1965. The company provided more than half the association's funding and exercised a great deal of control over its actions.[66] McGill University's Dr. John Corbett McDonald led this new study. JM's aim for the project was to "preserve the industry on which their business depends ... [and] avoid any undesirable publicity or any precipitate action by the USA or Canadian Federal Government which might be detrimental to the industry."[67] JM remained more concerned about bad publicity affecting profits than about the health of its employees. The company had dozens of confidential medical reports indicating that Jeffrey Mine employees were being placed at serious risk by working with such a dangerous mineral. Rather than fund better dust elimination equipment in Asbestos, the company chose to pay for medical reports to use as propaganda.

JM hoped that McDonald's study would eclipse Selikoff's and assure employees, shareholders, and the general public that pure chrysotile asbestos was safe. This was especially important when it came to Canada, since a 1965 study of one hundred randomly chosen autopsies at four Montreal hospitals showed a significant presence of asbestos fibres in 57 percent of the men examined and 34 percent of the women.[68] The air in all major Western cities was full of asbestos fibres because of the mineral's use in brake linings, cement, and general construction, all of which created dangerous dust. That the Canadian medical community had truly become interested in the mineral was significant in itself, but the fact that airborne fibres could contaminate people not directly involved with the industry was an earth-shaking discovery that could ruin the company. Meanwhile, the francophone medical community in Quebec was beginning to publish on incidences of mesothelioma in asbestos workers who had worked in the industry for over twenty years.[69] The company had to protect its interests in the province by proving that the people who worked at the Jeffrey Mine were healthy.

The industry's need for McDonald's results only increased as Selikoff continued to publish on the negative health effects of asbestos. Public opinion also began to turn against the mineral. QAMA admitted in their confidential meeting minutes that there was a direct link between asbestos and cancer and described Selikoff as "a healthy nemesis." Members worried that "we continue to receive an extremely bad press concerning the question of asbestos and health ... The time has come for us to produce some rebuttal ourselves, either in a general way or medically substantiated to the extent possible at this time."[70] Industry leaders were panicking and were looking for any evidence to prove that asbestos was not as bad as it seemed. Such panic was not only due to bad press. In July 1967, Liverpool dockworkers refused to unload shipments of the mineral unless it was packed in dust-proof containers, and in March 1968 Britain banned imports of crocidolite asbestos.[71]

Adding to these difficulties was the realization that if asbestos products were not shipped with warning labels, JM could be liable for any health problems the mineral caused. The American tobacco industry began putting warning labels on cigarettes in 1966, although these were initially quite vague. For reasons similar to those of the tobacco industry, especially the corporate fear of potential lawsuits, the company informed QAMA in 1968 that even if the rest of the industry voted against placing warning labels on shipments, JM would. The multilingual labels would read: "This product contains asbestos. Inhalation of asbestos dust over long periods of time may be harmful. Employees exposed to dust during use in application should be equipped with adequate personal protective devices."[72] This was not a severe warning, and it failed to mention cancer. It also failed to instill panic in Jeffrey Mine workers, who continued to refuse to wear respirators, operating within the risk parameters at the Jeffrey Mine as they understood them.[73]

Manufacturers all over the Western world objected to JM's labels and believed the warnings would cause unnecessary concern within their work-forces. A tile manufacturing company in Connecticut suggested that JM distribute an information pamphlet instead of the warning labels, and the Asbestos Fibre Importers Committee in England stated that "labour might refuse to handle asbestos unless packed in an impervious bag and probably insist on metal containers or fibre board drums" if the labels were visible to those in the shipping industry.[74] Complaints also arrived from manu-facturers in the Netherlands and Belgium: the labels caused financial trouble and emotional trauma, so JM should avoid the mistake of putting them on their shipments again.[75] These reactions show how strongly the people of Asbestos were internalizing the risks associated with the mineral their town was named for. Workers in Belgium were purportedly experi-encing emotional trauma, but those living next to the world's largest chrysotile asbestos mine remained calm. This put JM in a difficult position: the prospect of lawsuits against the company made the labels necessary, but warnings angered customers and agitated workers. In 1972, JM removed all warning labels from its Canadian products, on the basis that they were exempt from US regulations.[76] With an estimated 15,000 to 30,000 Can-adian jobs at risk if the industry collapsed, the company continued the "ignorance is bliss" policy that even company officials recognized was no longer working.

In 1968, the mills in Asbestos were finally refurbished with new dust-collecting technology. Only two years later, however, after learning that 175 of its Jeffrey Mine workers were suffering from asbestosis, company officials notified JM head office that the mill was too old to fix and that "we will have to live with the conditions until our new complex is in operation. We will encourage use of the Dustfoe 77 mask despite its prac-tical and personal comfort limitations [but d]isciplinary action to the point of layoff will be avoided."[77] Despite this managerial encouragement, Jeffrey Mine workers – only partly informed about the risks to their health – still refused to wear the uncomfortable respirators.

"Dust for Sale": 1971–83

In 1971, JM commissioned a study of asbestos-related cancers in local residents who did not work at the Jeffrey Mine. Large-scale environmental contamination had become a serious issue in the community. The study found a higher occurrence of bronchial cancer in Jeffrey Mine employees than among JM's American factory workers, and discovered that Asbestos residents faced a heightened risk of detrimental health consequences because of their proximity to the mine and the clouds of mineral dust that hovered over the town.[78] This undercut JM's claim that Canadian chrysotile was inert and led company officials to worry whether the community would be as tolerant of health risks as Jeffrey Mine employees had shown themselves to be.

By 1970, 114 of the 175 Jeffrey Mine workers suffering from asbestos-related disease, including cancer, had been informed of this fact by JM doctors.[79] Workers and their families were gaining vital information about what was happening to their bodies, but children continued to play in the dust that hovered over the community, writing their names in it as it settled on local parked cars.[80] Dust and risk had become part of community life. This did not mean that local residents liked it. Community members expressed their discontent with the fibrous dust clouds covering the town in a variety of ways. A headline in the local paper on July 13, 1971, read "Dust for Sale, Rue Bourbeau," and the accompanying article had an editorial cartoon that depicted a woman crossing the road covering her face against the blowing dust while her dog exclaimed, "If I had known that she wanted to cross the desert today, I wouldn't have gone out with her!"[81]

As dust became an increasingly difficult issue in Asbestos, the community was buffeted by changes that were transforming the global industry. Asbestos dust was now interesting health professionals, government agencies, and unions internationally. In 1969, Britain mandated a daily average exposure limit of two asbestos fibres per cubic centimetre (f/cc) for workers. This was an important step forward in occupational health regulation, but it also speaks to how hard it is to regulate the use of a hazardous material. In the late 1960s, asbestos was still of fundamental importance to industry, so rather than ban its use outright, regulators attempted to manage the risk. Such an approach failed to account for how specific jobs influenced exposure, or for the fact that someone exposed to 2 f/cc during a summer job could have a much lower risk of disease than someone who had worked in the factory for thirty years. In truth, all exposure to asbestos is harmful. This first regulation highlights the significant challenges of determining how workers are exposed to the hazardous mineral. During a time when they believed asbestos could be handled safely, regulators, industry heads, and employees themselves did not know how to factor in these variances.

Acknowledging the efforts of British regulatory bodies to reduce occupational exposure to asbestos, JM informed a doctor working for the Canadian government that an "internal standard" of 6 f/cc was being enforced at the Jeffrey Mine.[82] By 1971, the new US Occupational Safety and Health Administration (OSHA) had set a 5 f/cc industry-wide limit for worker exposure to asbestos dust, which legally required companies like JM to bring their operations up to this level of control. This should not have been an issue for a company that claimed its limit was 6 f/cc; however, an internal company survey of the dust levels in Jeffrey Mine operations in 1972 revealed that the mills had over 100 fibres of asbestos dust per cubic centimetre.[83] This was alarmingly high, and provides a good indication of what Jeffrey Mine mill employees coped with each day.

In 1976, OSHA reduced its daily average exposure limit for asbestos dust to the British standard of 2 f/cc.[84] When it was suggested that the company achieve 2 f/cc at the Jeffrey Mine, JM officials replied that it would be uneconomic and that it would lay off its employees rather than do so. JM was able to delay implementing the limit for years.

The dustiness of the Jeffrey Mine made its workers ideal subjects for the McGill study that JM and QAMA had been funding since 1965. McDonald found some incidences of pleural thickening in the lungs of his subjects at Asbestos, but he did not believe the mineral was at fault. He acknowledged that high levels of dust led directly to the development of mesothelioma, but he also claimed that cigarettes caused more lung damage than asbestos.[85] McDonald also studied 428 female employees and found that while they worked in extremely dusty areas, few of them had worked for more than ten years at the Jeffrey Mine, which resulted in fewer cases of disease. McDonald did not indicate whether he had looked for cancer of the breast or ovary.

JM received McDonald's conclusions positively because they mirrored Braun and Truan's report. He blamed the tobacco industry and the working class's supposed tendency to smoke cigarettes for heightened cancer rates among asbestos workers. The fact that McDonald was employed by McGill University gave the impression that his was an independent study of Quebec's asbestos workers. Even Selikoff hesitated to attack McDonald's conclusions. He disagreed with McDonald's results but observed rather tamely that the dust exposure levels for Canadian asbestos miners were apparently less than those for American insulation workers. Selikoff also accepted the idea that pure Canadian chrysotile might be less toxic than other types of asbestos, especially in its raw form.[86] Again favouring good publicity over the health of its employees, JM used McDonald's report to its fullest advantage.

In its 1973 newsletter to shareholders, JM claimed: "Much adverse, inaccurate publicity has surrounded the discussion of asbestos and human health. The mineral asbestos is unique and too valuable to do without ... As with many materials, asbestos can be harmful if not used properly."[87] Again, the problem was not with the mineral but rather with those who did not know how to work with it: they were responsible for their own asbestos-related disease, not JM. The company relied on McDonald's study and on the fact that it had spent over $20 million on improvements since 1962 to support its claims that the way JM handled asbestos made the mineral completely safe. The newsletter also claimed that dust counts in the company's manufacturing plants were below 5 f/cc. This statement was misleading and focused solely on JM factories in the United States. It also avoided any specific mention of the mill at the Jeffrey Mine, which continued to have dust counts above 100 f/cc.

McDonald further aided JM's claims that the mineral was safe by publishing in the *Canadian Medical Association Journal* in 1973. There he stated that there was no significantly higher rate of occurrence of mesothelioma among asbestos workers than among the province as a whole between 1960 and 1970. Although he conceded that some victims of mesothelioma had been domestically exposed to asbestos through their interactions with family members who worked in the industry, he insisted that this did not mean the mineral was especially deadly or that it was the only cause of the disease.[88] His paper suggested that the asbestos industry had been the victim of faulty medical reports that blamed the mineral for any disease that occurred in those who worked with it.

Hard on the heels of McDonald's publication, JM officials hosted a QAMA meeting with other international asbestos manufacturing companies. Confidential minutes from that meeting suggest that although McDonald's report had bought the industry some time to regroup after being so thoroughly attacked in the medical community, the press, and the American courts, officials knew this calm would not last long. One official stated that the "all important problem ... is how to deal with Selikoff ... Within the Industry, Johns-Manville is the only Company with sound acknowledged expertise... The battle is still continuing and [the] Industry needs help."[89] JM was important to industry leaders because of its control over the world's largest and "safest" chrysotile mine and its international reach through trade and manufacturing networks.

Another advantage JM had, according to QAMA, was that "the question of asbestos & health was not as big a problem in Canada as in the USA. Besides, the audience is mostly confined to Quebec and more in the English than in the French Press. It seems that the French media have never tackle[d] too strongly the asbestos & health problem. It should be pointed out, however, that the release of the McDonald report received excellent press coverage."[90] Because JM's workforce was mainly unilingual francophone, industry leaders felt there was a safe buffer between them and damning medical reports about the health effects of asbestos. Furthermore, aside from LeDoux's 1949 exposé and Pelletier's coverage of the resulting strike in Asbestos, QAMA's observations were correct; the francophone press in Quebec did not concern itself about health issues affecting the workers in one of the province's most lucrative industries. Both LeDoux and Pelletier moved on to other issues, and nobody took their place. English Canada had little interest in small-town Quebec, although the Ontario government would eventually launch a Royal Commission to study the health effects of asbestos on its workers. French Canadians were caught up in issues of Québécois nationalism and sovereignty, which dominated the francophone media and the medical community.[91] For the time being, at least, the industry was flying under the radar in Quebec.

Canada's English media were a larger problem for JM. Reporters knew about Selikoff's speeches and about reports on the damaging effects of asbestos. In 1974, CBC radio interviewed McDonald and repeatedly asked him whether his study was funded by the asbestos industry. After initially claiming that only McGill supported his work, he eventually admitted that QAMA had donated a significant amount of research money to the university.[92] When the *New York Times* ran an article condemning McDonald's study because of its links to the asbestos industry, McDonald threatened to sue the newspaper's editor for libel, insisting that although QAMA had provided funds for the study, he was acting on the request of the Canadian government, not the industry. The international attention focused on Quebec's asbestos mines soon led to a resurgence of interest in the industry among the francophone medical community. One report in *La vie médicale au Canada français* indicated that mesothelioma occurrences were 1 in 10,000 for the general population but 1 in 10 for those working in Quebec's asbestos industry.[93]

These numbers were alarming, and JM's pretense that the Jeffrey Mine was the perfect example of health began to crumble – as did profits. In response, JM's new Health, Safety and Environment vice-president Paul Kotin sent filmmaker Walter Cooper to Asbestos in May 1975 to make a pro-industry documentary called "Asbestos and Health." Cooper wrote to Kotin that on arrival,

> the bagging operation on the main floor was shocking. There were accumulations of dust everywhere. It took more than an hour to clean up one bagging unit of visible dust before filming. At another bag unit, I noticed an ankle-high accumulation of fiber, which was being shovelled into an open cart for disposal by a worker, who was not wearing a respirator.[94]

Cooper's observations echoed those of John Knox, the British doctor who had inspected operations at the Jeffrey Mine in 1952. The fact that dust levels remained alarmingly high after more than twenty years demonstrates just how ineffectual JM's efforts to reduce dust in the mill had been, despite the company's awareness of the severe health risks associated with asbestos. Cooper's report also suggests how accustomed employees had become to being surrounded by dust, even after company doctors had started informing them of their asbestos-related disease.

Cooper's observations offer a rare glimpse into the Jeffrey Mine in 1975. According to his account: "Fiber continued to spill from the bags onto the floor, where other workers tracked through it ... I saw a [quality control] man at the bagging operation open at least four bags, grab a handful of fiber, throw it into an open plate, and then break it apart and swish it around. He did not wear a respirator."[95] Cooper was astounded at the amount of dust in the air at the Jeffrey Mine and had to stop filming three times to clean his equipment. He noted that the mill he was filming in had been closed for repairs and had just completed its weekly two-hour cleaning session, done mostly with brooms, which did a better job of stirring up clouds of dust than eliminating them. When the filming was over, Cooper and his cameramen found their clothes, bodies, and hair – as well as their cars in the parking lot – covered with dust.

Jeffrey Mine workers were aware of the dangerous mineral dust they worked with each day, but also limited in terms of how they could address their exposure. Their union could lobby for better dust control measures at the mine, and workers could strike if JM refused to provide them. But workers were reluctant to launch this type of labour action because the industry was increasingly unstable, with health and safety lawsuits being brought against American asbestos companies by workers in the United States. Employees could move away from Asbestos and find work in a different industry, but this would not have prevented the progression of asbestos-related disease in their bodies. Also, moving away from the community – and industry – after generations of life and labour there was easier said than done. As historical geographer David Robertson has shown in *Hard as the Rock Itself,* living in a town devoted to mining "reinforces individual and social-group identities … [and] reminds them that they are members of a strong, hardworking, and persevering communit[y]. In fact, the physical and economic challenges of mining life often produce communities with a marked ability to endure."[96]

Soon after Cooper's visit to Asbestos, Health and Welfare Canada released its first study on asbestos-related disease. It showed that Ontario, which had a large automobile manufacturing industry that made heavy use of asbestos, had 69 cases of mesothelioma between 1960 and 1970, and that Quebec had at least 102 in the same decade. It concluded that even if chrysotile was safer than other types of asbestos fibre, "definite health hazards exist in the Canadian workplace due to high levels of occupational exposures to asbestos together with inadequate health surveillance and protection."[97] By 1975, the Canadian government knew that asbestos workers were at risk. It also knew that companies like JM were not addressing the issue adequately. Yet that same year, JM assured its shareholders that occupational and community exposure to asbestos dust was not a significant issue.[98] No one in government moved to change the company's approach to occupational health and safety. Yet the company finally made respirators mandatory if exposure was above 2 f/cc.[99] The respirators designed for this type of filtration, however, were useless in environments like the Jeffrey Mine's mill, where the concentration of dust was so high that the filters clogged immediately, making it even more difficult to breathe.

When health concerns led Thetford workers to strike in 1975, the employees at Asbestos followed them but kept their dispute to wages.[100] Although Jeffrey Mine workers refused to indict JM for safety violations, publicity on the negative health effects of asbestos was rapidly increasing. In the United States, the EPA became involved as American mothers began to fear for the safety of their children who attended schools insulated with asbestos. Hoping to gain credibility or perhaps some control over the situation, in 1976 JM funded a program designed by Selikoff to find ways to detect mesothelioma early enough to cure it. A year later the company introduced a "no smoking" policy for all its workers because "research shows that asbestos workers who do not smoke cigarettes have no greater incidence of lung cancer than is found in the general population. Asbestos workers who do smoke, however, have an incidence of lung cancer that is 92 times greater than asbestos workers who don't smoke."[101] The tobacco industry and the assumed habits of the working class were once again a convenient scapegoat, but the policy had little effect on how outsiders perceived operations at the Jeffrey Mine. The Beaudry Inquiry convened in 1976 to look into the health of the province's asbestos workers after the Thetford strike, and was appalled at the levels of dust workers were exposed to each day.[102] Governments were beginning to take notice of the health problem in the asbestos industry, but loose regulations were blamed, not the inherent danger of the mineral.

Echoing this approach, JM's Health, Safety and Environment vice-president Paul Kotin wrote: "If the division cannot complete the environmental clean-up of this textile operation, then serious consideration should be given to shutting down the operation [in Asbestos]. The Jeffrey Textile Plant is an embarrassment as it does not meet [JM's] standards and has not met them for a good number of years."[103] Jeffrey Mine operations could not be shut down because they provided most of JM's raw mineral and were the keystone of the company's defence against claims that asbestos was dangerous. By November 1977, the company had made the wearing of protective clothing and respirators mandatory in areas with a fibre count above 1.2 f/cc.[104] This was well within the 2 f/cc new limit set by the Quebec government the previous year. As a result, a 1978 CBC Radio report on Quebec's asbestos industry left the Jeffrey Mine out and instead spawned headlines such as, "Véritable génocide à Thetford," which had not reached these relatively low levels of exposure.[105]

Despite increasingly negative publicity in Canada and a growing number of occupational health lawsuits launched by its American workers, JM continued to pose as an industry leader in occupational safety. In its 1980 edition of *JM Today*, the company provided a "Special Asbestos Update" in response to rising global criticism of asbestos sales to countries in the developing world. The article claimed that JM refused to sell its products to countries and places that would not uphold the strict health regulations placed on the American asbestos industry. It also denied that the company had ever withheld damning medical reports from its employees, and denounced the idea that asbestos did more harm than good. JM claimed that its products were essential in developing countries that required shelter and reliable water and sewer systems because "providing these with asbestos cement products does not require sophisticated technology. It requires for the most part simply the importation of asbestos fiber – a material much less costly than substitute building materials such as steel, imported wood, or petroleum-based products."[106]

In the same issue of the magazine, the town of Asbestos was featured as the source of all the potential good that could come from JM products. The magazine profiled Norman Chartier, a mill supervisor who had worked at the Jeffrey Mine for four decades and who hoped to boost the image of asbestos. Chartier hinted at the character of the community when he stated that no job was 100 percent safe, but "if a man uses common sense on the job and follows the rules set down for his protection, he's more apt to get into trouble when he's not working."[107] This was the type of information the company wanted its employees to believe and publicize. Chartier also dismissed recent negative accounts of the industry as meaningless propaganda based on long outdated information. He stated that the "enormous effort and energy devoted by the company over the past several years in protecting workers' health is beginning to pay off ... If you believe everything you read in the newspapers or watch on television about asbestos, then there's no future for our industry."[108]

In Chartier's opinion, he had lived "the good life" in Asbestos thanks to the mineral, and "under today's conditions, I'd encourage people to work in this industry. As a matter of fact, if I were starting all over again, I wouldn't hesitate – I'd apply for the same job again."[109] Chartier asserted that he was not worried about his health although he had worked in one of the dustiest areas of the mine since 1936. His life and the risks it entailed had been what the residents of Asbestos had expected and accepted for generations. While JM now informed employees of their illnesses when they were discovered, officials maintained that the company had done no wrong by keeping reports secret in the past because Asbestos was a company town with few jobs and scant prospects beyond the mine.[110]

A year later, in 1981, the company released a pamphlet titled "Asbestos, Health and Johns-Manville." This attributed recently identified asbestos-related diseases to a lack of knowledge decades earlier and insisted that no new cases would develop now that the company was aware of the risks.[111] Yet, the first reported fatal case of asbestosis had been in Britain in 1906.[112] The first civil lawsuit launched by a JM employee against the company was in 1929.[113] False though they were, JM's claims were good public relations. So too were statements by members of the Canadian medical community that, while carcinogenic, chrysotile was less dangerous than other types of asbestos and that working with the mineral was equivalent to smoking only three or four cigarettes a week.[114]

The support of the Canadian medical community was important because it legitimized JM's claims to past ignorance and drew public attention away from the issue. The Canadian medical community – both anglophone and francophone – had been exposed to international reports detailing the epidemiology of asbestos-related disease but had chosen not to investigate further. The fact that knowledge of the risks associated with asbestos came from the company rather than from independent researchers meant that JM shaped the community's understanding of the dangers the mineral posed. The detrimental health effects of the mineral could no longer be completely denied, but the way the people of Asbestos intertwined their sense of self with their sense of place, combined with the process by which they were made aware of the mineral's risk, meant they remained committed to the industry.

For all the support it received in Asbestos, JM continued to be plagued by litigation in the United States, where product liability laws made the company vulnerable to individual lawsuits that could result in multimillion-dollar verdicts and bad press around the world. Relying on the supposed good health of Jeffrey Mine employees was no longer enough. In 1982, unable to meet the rising costs of litigation, and anticipating 52,000 new lawsuits averaging $40,000 each, JM filed for bankruptcy.[115] The company left the Jeffrey Mine in 1983 after having been an important, although controversial, presence in Asbestos for more than half a century. Still, the provincial government and the people of Asbestos remained committed to the industry. Under René Lévesque's Parti Québécois, the Quebec government nationalized the industry, making it a state entity, and eventually subsidized the town. Furthermore, a new public company named JM Asbestos took over the Jeffrey Mine.

Nationalization effectively blocked any outside inquiries into the health of the workers in Asbestos. This began a trend in which the provincial and federal governments supported the industry by doing what JM could no longer do, which was deny damning medical reports, ignore the welfare of community members, refuse to properly label shipments of asbestos to other countries, and sell the mineral to developing nations. Some of the town's almost 8,000 citizens left to seek more stable, healthy employment, but most remained. The people of Asbestos should not have had to choose between their jobs and their health, but that is just what many had to do. The environmental reality of Asbestos – it was built atop of a massive asbestos deposit, nestled next to a giant opencast mine – was such that there was very little that townspeople could do for work that did not involve the industry.

Government subsidies and JM's manipulation of medical evidence have been the focus of academic studies and media reports, but more significant has been the near total reliance of the local community on the global asbestos industry and the risks this dependence encouraged them to take.

8

Altered Authority, 1949–83

I N 2004, AND AGAIN in 2011, Asbestos and Canada made international headlines at the UN's Rotterdam Convention when government officials prevented chrysotile asbestos from being placed on the Prior Informed Consent list of dangerous minerals, which would have hindered trade in the fibre. The government justified this manoeuvre by stating that asbestos is safe, "provided it is manufactured, handled with care, and exposures to dust are stringently prevented or controlled to low levels."[1] Officials failed to mention the danger of the mineral in its raw form, and the government made no effort to ensure that proper health and safety regulations were upheld in the developing countries to which it sold asbestos. This was not without its price. Two historians of the global asbestos trade, Jock McCulloch and Geoffrey Tweedale, write that one of the major constants in the history of the industry has been "the malevolent role played by Canada in promoting asbestos use in the developing world. Canada is a member of the G8 and it carries some influence on the global stage. Its industry and government, backed by a sophisticated scientific community, have used their access to elite forums, including the WHO [World Health Organization] and the WTO [World Trade Organization], to promote asbestos."[2] Russia was the other major supplier of asbestos to markets in developing nations, and Canada's position in Rotterdam and its reputation as an "international Boy Scout"[3] led American asbestos scholar Barry Castleman to reflect: "If the only people saying it's good are the Russians, we can deal with that. Canada saying it's good makes it more complicated."[4]

THE STRUGGLE FOR LIFE: 1949–52

This chapter explores how the people of Asbestos worked in tandem with government officials to support the industry and maintain their community and the Jeffrey Mine despite the health risks associated with the latter between 1949 and 1983. When the strike of 1949 ended in July, the local paper printed the agreement so that everyone would be aware of the terms of settlement. Although some issues were reserved for arbitration, the government recertified the union, and JM allowed striking workers to return to their jobs as quickly as production rates allowed.[5] The company also agreed to expand its underground mining operations and to take on one hundred more employees. The townspeople of Asbestos were jubilant: it seemed that jobs and prospects had been restored. However, JM president Lewis H. Brown was adamant that they not conclude that they had "won" the five-month battle that had just taken place. He sent a letter to each employee detailing the terms of the agreement and making it clear that the company, not the working class of the community, had been victorious.[6] Brown's letter explained – as had another he sent to the lead settlement arbitrator, Archbishop of Quebec Maurice Roy – that the company would be reducing employment levels at the mill and that the "reduction in employment would have taken place even had there been no strike at all." A global recession was identified as the basic cause of persisting unemployment in Asbestos; it was, said Brown, "still the heart of the problem and everyone there must be made to understand the facts."[7]

Actually, international demand for asbestos was high after five months without production from Asbestos. Brown also misled when he said that all the workers except those facing criminal charges would be "put back to their occupation" at their 1948 wages, when what he meant was that they could be assigned *any* job at the Jeffrey Mine rather than their former positions. Strikebreakers had by then taken many of the positions originally filled by strikers.[8] Brown was determined that the people of Asbestos understand and accept their defeat.

In July, only 260 of the 2,100 workers who had gone on strike were taken back at the Jeffrey Mine. Over the strike's duration, union workers had lost an average of $1,066 each in wages,[9] and those who were not rehired were outraged that strikebreakers, mostly from outside Asbestos, were working their jobs. After receiving Brown's letter, groups of unemployed union men roamed the streets late into the night, throwing rocks through the windows of homes where strikebreakers or JM sympathizers lived. They also assaulted any "scabs" they encountered, and burned down a garage in Tingwick, where many of the still employed strikebreakers lived.[10] Police received a flurry of calls from Tingwick residents afraid of the mob, who were angry with the situation and anxious about the future.

JM responded by increasing police patrols at the Jeffrey Mine to ensure that the disgruntled men would not attack company operations. The mine was firmly under JM's control but remained a potential battleground. Denying bias in favour of the company, the local newspaper tried to calm the people of Asbestos by suggesting that it was time to move on and that enough had been written about the conflict, which now needed to be forgotten.[11] By contrast, the Quebec press and unions compared every new labour dispute in the province to the one in Asbestos.

Post-strike Asbestos was radically different from its predecessor. Townspeople worried about how poor industrial relations and power struggles between JM and the workers would harm the community. In August 1949, a local resident named Bertrand McNeil captured the uncertainty and unease prevalent in Asbestos when he wrote to Quebec Minister of Labour Antonio Barrette:

> I'm 20 years old, I've had a year and a half of service [at the Jeffrey Mine] and I need to work. I've had no bad relations with the company. I would like to know if they are going to take all of us back or if we're waiting for nothing. My father has a large family and I'm the only one who can help them. I'm paying for my 16 year old brother to become a priest.[12]

McNeil's concern for his family demonstrates how much townspeople depended on JM for employment and how hard it must have been for these large families to survive during the strike. In its reply, the arbitration board working on the strike settlement told McNeil that unemployment in Asbestos would end soon, but gave no definite date to ease his worries.[13]

McNeil was one of dozens in Asbestos in 1949 who aspired to nothing more than a life of stable employment at the Jeffrey Mine. The essential qualities of his letter were echoed in September 1949 by Madame Eugène Tourigny, who also wrote to Barrette: "You may find me demanding, but you know I have a mother's heart and when I see my children without work, it gives me great sorrow to see strikebreakers making the women and children of the strikers suffer so … It's a great tragedy for Asbestos."[14] The same letter claimed that strikebreakers had developed a hubris that led them to intimidate local women and children.

JM's slow re-employment of striking workers drove a wedge deeper between the company and the community. In October 1949, town council began negotiations with Shawinigan Water and Power to install power lines in the newer sections of town[15] and acquired trucks to install power poles – responsibilities previously left to JM. At year's end, both JM and the local newspaper expressed a wish for peaceful company-community relations,[16] but many former strikers remained unemployed, and everyone worried about future contract negotiations. As 1950 began, American Karl V. Lindell replaced G.K. Foster as president of C-JM. Foster had been wildly unpopular in Asbestos since his involvement in the provincial police's brutality at the Hotel Iroquois during the strike, and Lindell struck a conciliatory note when he spoke to townspeople of his hopes for the future and his commitment to learn French. Even today, the town remembers Lindell fondly as someone who brought a new attitude of cooperation and consideration to Asbestos.[17]

Lindell's approach provided an opening for the town council. In February 1950, council demanded that JM find work for those Asbestos residents left unemployed because of the strike.[18] If Lindell was sincere in his commitment to the community, he needed to return the formerly striking workers to their jobs at the Jeffrey Mine. Indeed, most of them were taken back by April.

In March 1950, the collective agreement between the workers and JM that had been pending since December 1948 was finally signed. Workers received a 10 cent per hour raise, one additional paid holiday, and two weeks of vacation after being employed at the Jeffrey Mine for three years.[19] Left unaddressed were the major issues of land use, dust control, and the desire for employees to have a say in company promotions.

The community saw the new contract as an achievement, but its ratification revealed how desperate workers were for work, and many worried about how the conflict and settlement had affected the town's image. The press continued to compare new labour disputes in Quebec to the asbestos strike, and Duplessis used the violence of the conflict to reinforce his anti-communist Padlock Law and limit the power of unions in Quebec. When Archbishop of Montreal Joseph Charbonneau was removed from his position and forced into a West Coast retirement in February 1950, the international press believed it was because of the role he had played in the strike.[20] Many speculated that Sherbrooke's bishop, Philippe Desranleau, would follow Charbonneau for similar reasons, but his untimely death prevented it. The strike was becoming part of Quebec's political culture, which conferred on the people of Asbestos an influence they neither sought nor fully understood.

Cultural changes aside, the asbestos industry continued to boom despite the freeze the strike had enforced on it. Notwithstanding Brown's claims about the global recession, in April 1950 C-JM announced it would be sharing a surplus of $70,000 with its employees, almost all of whom had been hired back.[21] This profit-sharing gesture was part of Lindell's new approach to industrial relations in Asbestos, but despite the positive feelings it generated, a referendum in May authorized the town to spend $100,000 to attract new industries.[22] The unemployment problem following the strike had illustrated what many people already knew: that it was dangerous to rely on one industry and a single employer. No major new industry ever came to Asbestos, however, reinforcing the idea that without asbestos, the community would die.

Company-community relations continued to improve under Lindell's management. In 1950 the company celebrated for the first time St-Jean-Baptiste Day in June and Labour Day in September with its employees and their families. Union heads were present, and Father Camirand gave a picnic mass. Workers and company officials had come to terms with the power each held in the community and were able to coexist because of this understanding. Twenty-nine new members of the Quarter-Century Club were inducted in 1950, bringing the total number of employees who had worked at the Jeffrey Mine for at least twenty-five years up to 205 – longer than most JM officials had been in Asbestos.[23] By October, almost half the town's population worked at the Jeffrey Mine, matching the pre-strike employment rate. Authority in Asbestos was shared among the workers, JM, and town officials because they depended on one another for survival, but Asbestos purchased its own snowploughs so that it would not have to rely on JM to clear the winter streets, as it had in the past.[24]

This balance was maintained into 1951, when JM and the union signed a new collective agreement with little dispute. Workers received a 15 percent wage increase, a bonus for those on night shifts, one more paid holiday each year, and a social security plan that both JM and its employees paid into equally. These were significant accomplishments. The company also promised to rehire within three months all of those who had been unemployed since the strike. These harmonious relations led the local paper to write "All's quiet, they say, in Asbestos."[25] In May, JM opened Jeffrey Mine operations to more than 3,500 community members to celebrate the 70th anniversary of the pit.[26] On Labour Day, Lindell's address to the community included this observation: "Work, it's the struggle for life. The Creator has surrounded us with riches that He wants us to exploit for our benefit."[27] Work, religion, and the mine formed the foundations for Asbestos.

While these three pillars were central to the community, the town of Asbestos became central to Quebec's labour movement. In the summer of 1951, seventy-five union heads representing miners throughout Quebec held their annual meeting in Asbestos. Local workers maintained faith in the strength of unions. The CTCC had convinced JM to drop the charges against local union heads Rodolphe Hamel and Armande Larivée, along with nineteen others, for their roles in the riot of May 1949. The union was also instrumental in convincing the company to rehire the last striking worker who had not been taken back and to return all workers to their original positions.[28] Thanks to Lindell's public initiatives, JM and its employees were on excellent terms in the early 1950s. The same could not be said for the town and the province. Asbestos had long supported the Union Nationale by electing Mayor Albert Goudreau as its provincial representative, but his popularity had dissipated by 1949, and he lost in the next municipal election. Goudreau remained committed to Duplessis and to representing the people of Asbestos, but he was harassed by townspeople when he campaigned in the 1952 election, which he also lost.[29] They had not forgotten how the government had sent provincial police to the community, nor Goudreau's ineffectiveness in sending them away.

Local support for candidates in the Quebec election of 1952 was shown in much the same way as support for the 1949 strike in Asbestos: through church alliances. On July 3, Goudreau held a Union Nationale rally with Minister of Industry and Commerce Paul Beaulieu in St-Isaac-Jogues, the church that many local residents had boycotted during the strike because its priest was against the conflict. Hundreds of disgruntled townspeople attended, and heard Goudreau ask whether things would be better if the community returned to a time before Duplessis. Only one of those in attendance was brave enough to yell, "Talk to us about the strike!" Beaulieu condescendingly replied, "The strike is a settled affair, young man," which only further angered the crowd.[30] Despite harmonious company-community relations, the strike was not a settled affair in Asbestos.

Liberal candidate Émilien Lafrance did not make the same mistake as Goudreau. The Liberals held their rally at St-Aimé, the church of choice for the workers during the strike and still a politically charged place because of the police violence there in May 1949. In his speech, Lafrance dared

Duplessis to come to Asbestos and say that he truly sympathized with the working class. Carrier Fortin, a CTCC lawyer, also spoke and said that Duplessis had proven his loathing for workers, and if they "returned him to power, they will be in an open conflict with the government ... But there is one day every 4 or 5 years where the workers are the masters, where they are the most strong."[31] Election Day was the time when the people of Asbestos could demonstrate their collective strength after being humbled by the 1949 strike. The Liberals knew that Asbestos was theirs to lose.

The Duplessis government was re-elected in almost every riding in Quebec. Asbestos was one of the few places outside Montreal where the Liberals won a seat.[32] The Union Nationale dropped 17 percent in the popular vote; the Liberals increased their presence in the legislature from eight seats to 23. The people of Asbestos celebrated the results of the election in the streets of the town and in the basement of St-Aimé, happy to have won this small battle.

"A Remarkable Personality Is Revealed": 1953–72

The town of Asbestos continued to vote Liberal until 1970. Although Duplessis visited in 1954 to open a new mill, townspeople did not forgive him, as they had JM. Company-community relations in Asbestos continued to be good, with JM now providing a minimum pension of $110 per month for its retired employees.[33] The company and its workers had come to an understanding about the important roles both played in the success of the community and the industry. JM ran public relations campaigns stressing the importance of Asbestos to the global industry. In May 1955, its employee newsletter further emphasized the importance of JM workers in an article in which a son questioned his father about the value of his job. The father replied: "My son, it is true that I wear workers [sic] clothes, and that I have dirty hands. But, don't be ashamed to tell your friends that asbestos fibre, which I help produce, plays a role in both national and international industry."[34] While it was a fictional conversation, this article highlighted some prominent characteristics of Asbestos. Jeffrey Mine workers were proud of the role they played in the global industry, and it was common in the community for sons to follow fathers into employment at the mine.

Articles like this spoke to issues that concerned the community. They supported the idea that labour was valuable and that jobs at the Jeffrey Mine offered an appealing future for the community's children. A group

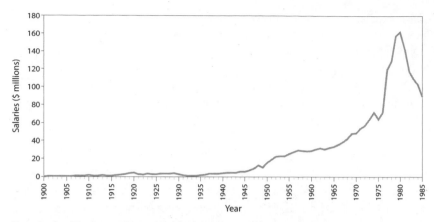

FIGURE 20　Total pay given to Quebec's asbestos workers, 1900–85
Source: Data provided the Province of Quebec (http://www.mern.gouv.qc.ca/mines/
desminesetdeshommes/index.jsp#annexe), compiled by Marc Vallières

of intellectuals from outside Asbestos overlooked these local issues, however, and assigned different importance to the community. Future prime
minister of Canada Pierre Trudeau's *La grève de l'amiante*, released in 1956,
detailed how the 1949 strike in Asbestos had radically changed Quebec
society and politics, partly because of the resource's importance to the
provincial economy. Trudeau was especially effective at using the strike
to shape a vision of Quebec that he treasured, one that included French
Canadians rebelling against their foreign employers and claiming their
natural resource industries for themselves.[35] Maurice Sauvé wrote the only
chapter that actually studied the community in detail; in it, he acknowledged the harmonious industrial relations in Asbestos since the conflict.
He also showed that many of the demands the workers had made during
the 1949 strike had been implemented, making JM employees the best-
paid miners in the country (see Figure 20).[36]

　　But Sauvé's chapter was overshadowed by Trudeau's introduction and
conclusion, which signalled radical changes in Quebec's social and political
culture. Intellectuals avidly debated Trudeau's ideas in newspapers, journals, and academic circles throughout the province.[37] A 1999 local history
of the town addressed these sentiments, stating that Trudeau and his con-
tributors had seen what they wanted to see in the strike and were not
concerned with the actual results of the conflict. With this local history,
townspeople wanted "to bring more attention to the local debate, seen
in how the conflict shaped the collective conscience of the people of
Asbestos."[38]

The strike was deeply personal for the community, and removing it from its local context put their painful memories on display. But it would be Trudeau's book, not the strike itself, that would influence how the province viewed Asbestos – and Quebec's other resource industry workers – in the decades to come. Townspeople did not see themselves as at the forefront of radical political change, and they did not want the notoriety that came with that perception. The community remained focused on working the Jeffrey Mine. Local residents also became increasingly isolationist, and tensions emerged with the small fraction of JM's workforce that came from surrounding towns.

The strikebreakers hired in 1949 had turned the local population against anyone at the Jeffrey Mine who was not from Asbestos. Although it had no authority to do so, council lobbied JM to stop hiring workers from outside the community and tried to encourage nonlocal employees to move into Asbestos by offering free rent for a year and a special discount at certain local stores.[39] This amounted to a sharp reversal of the community's 1927 ruling that levied an extra tax on those who had not lived in the town for at least a year.

Despite their best efforts to focus solely on local affairs, the people of Asbestos could not remain aloof from the political discourse of the province. Ten years after Trudeau's book was published, Pierre Vallières of the Front de libération du Québec (FLQ), a political terrorist group in the province committed to Quebec sovereignty, wrote *Nègres blancs d'Amérique (White Niggers of America)*. In his inflammatory book, Vallières rooted the ideals of the province's terrorist movement of the 1960s and 1970s in the 1949 strike.[40] This included the FLQ kidnapping of politicians, one of whom was murdered, and the planting of bombs in mailboxes. Vallières argued that workers had taken control of Asbestos and "refused to obey their leaders," in much the same way that the FLQ refused to obey laws that subjugated French Canadians and "aroused the people against the monarch of 'the great darkness'" of oppression.[41] Vallières's gross misrepresentation of the strike and the people of Asbestos exceeded even Trudeau's. Yet both books continued to influence outside perceptions of the community.

During the provincial election campaign of 1960, Asbestos became a political football, with Liberal leader Jean Lesage running against the Union Nationale's Antonio Barrette, who had been labour minister during the 1949 strike. Lesage attacked Barrette by invoking the labour dispute and repeatedly accused Barrette of holing up in Bermuda with JM officials "during the bloody asbestos strike."[42] Lesage's accusation was reported throughout the province, and Barrette had to respond to the newly symbolic nature of Asbestos and the strike. The Liberals soundly defeated the Union Nationale.

The 1949 strike – and the community of Asbestos, in particular – were constantly referred to while political changes swept Quebec in the 1960s. Rooted in this change was a commitment by the new Lesage government to gain control of the province's vast natural resources so that Quebec would truly become "Maîtres chez nous" – that is, "masters in our own house." When Premier Lesage visited Asbestos in 1962, he told townspeople that it was time for French Canadians to control the province's profitable resource industries.[43] This referred not only to a change in management at places like the Jeffrey Mine, but also to a change in how natural resource industries were run in the province, with the government becoming the key stakeholder.

JM was less concerned about the outcome of the political changes in the province than it might have been, because officials had a larger issue to deal with: health. International awareness of asbestos-related disease was growing, and at Lindell's insistence, QAMA aligned itself with the federal government in 1965, hoping to block any regulations that would hinder production.[44] Lindell also spoke to the people of Asbestos, urging them to work with the company to fight against the mineral's tarnished image. The industry's workers, who continued to lack a comprehensive understanding of how the mineral was affecting their health, were to become its greatest defenders.

Worker support became increasingly important when Pierre Trudeau, Jean Marchand, and Gérard Pelletier all won federal seats in 1968, with Trudeau as prime minister. All three had been present in Asbestos during the 1949 strike and had helped turn the conflict into a political symbol. In response, JM officials expressed concern to QAMA that the new Quebec premier, Daniel Johnson, "might try to be more friendly with labour, should Trudeau and Marchand become the leaders in Ottawa." If that happened, "as a result industry could be affected."[45] Trudeau, Pelletier, and especially Marchand, the former CTCC secretary, knew of the health risks of asbestos, and they knew how the French Canadian working class had been treated by foreign companies in the past.

JM officials reacted to the election by going on the offensive and meeting with union leaders and town council to negotiate the rebuilding of a factory that the company was demolishing because of health violations.[46] Helping JM in this was the fact that the people of Asbestos were not full participants in the socio-political revolution then sweeping Quebec. They

supported the CTCC becoming the Confédération des syndicats nationaux (CSN) and breaking away from the Catholic Church in 1960, as well
as the CSN demanding that French become the official workplace language in Quebec. But Jeffrey Mine workers gradually lost faith in the
increasingly radical CSN and voted to break with the union in 1972.[47] A
few weeks later, the local union joined the more moderate Centrale des
syndicates démocratiques (CSD).

Becoming Spectacular, 1973–83

Content with their more moderate union, at the end of 1972 the workers
at the Jeffrey Mine produced 13 percent of the global supply of asbestos
and shipped 94 percent of it to more than seventy countries.[48] Because
asbestos companies were increasingly worried that the health effects of the
mineral would negatively affect trade, they formed the Asbestos Information Committee. This was an international association with members from
Canada, the United States, and the United Kingdom whose mandate was
to promote the industry, although QAMA did not think the Canadian
industry was as threatened as those in other countries.[49]

Notwithstanding QAMA's assurances, the Canadian industry was under
threat in the 1970s. Sensing this, JM rapidly expanded its extraction efforts
at the Jeffrey Mine in order to get as much mineral as possible to market
before the industry collapsed. Increased extraction levels also meant fast-
tracked expansion plans for the Jeffrey Mine, as well as heightened tensions
between the local population and the company. A special edition of the
local newspaper, marking the seventy-fifth anniversary of the town, me-
morialized all the neighbourhoods that had been destroyed by the expanding Jeffrey Mine. It also dedicated three pages to the 1949 strike, noting
that the conflict had been the most dramatic in the history of Quebec
trade unionism and had been deeply engraved in the hearts and spirits of
the townspeople.[50] The people of Asbestos might disapprove of those outside the community appropriating their past for political ends, but they
had grown accustomed to that past's symbolic value. The paper explained
that because of the major political and religious figures involved in the
strike, the town had "become something spectacular."[51]

The same special edition featured letters from Pierre Trudeau congratu-
lating the community on its anniversary and from Gérard Pelletier reflecting
on his experiences during the strike. Trudeau reiterated his 1956 interpretation of the labour dispute, observing that the townspeople had a remarkable

faith in the future and possessed a courage and a determination that the entire country admired. [52] Photographs of Trudeau, Pelletier, and Marchand in Asbestos were displayed throughout the special edition, which also included a feature on René Lévesque as head of the new sovereignist Parti Québécois (PQ). Lévesque had held his party's regional convention in Asbestos in 1974, and the paper asserted that any politician who wanted votes in Quebec had to visit the community and sympathize with its working class.[53] This was a daring claim to make as the industry began to collapse.

The political attention Asbestos received in the 1970s gave townspeople the impression that the industry and the community were less threatened by negative global opinion than they once had been. Driven by confidence, 2,000 Jeffrey Mine workers struck in February 1975 to gain a wage increase and health insurance. They also wanted a guarantee that their shifts would be at least eight hours long each day; this was a response to cutbacks in manpower as sophisticated machines and crumbling markets made employees redundant.[54] Both sides compromised and resolved the dispute for the sake of production.

With the election of Lévesque's PQ government in 1976, the "maîtres chez nous" movement gained new purchase in Quebec. Asbestos town council articulated this awareness when it stated that the French language needed to be reborn in Quebec in order to influence the provincial economy in such a way that profits did not immediately go to foreign interests.[55] This was an important stance for the people of Asbestos to take, given their bicultural heritage and long reliance on an American company and global industry.

But the terms of concern changed when Lévesque targeted asbestos as the next resource industry for nationalization. The industry was suffering, but it was still profitable, and the 1949 strike had become such a powerful symbol of modernity and strength in the province that the PQ found the industry especially desirable. The government created the Bureau de l'amiante in 1977 to study the economic potential and health risks of asbestos. Believing that the benefits outweighed the risks, the PQ began the process of nationalization. JM officials were wary of all this but admitted that nationalization would create 7,000 to 8,000 new jobs once government capital was invested in the manufacture of asbestos products.[56] In the end, 2,500 Jeffrey Mine workers voted in favour of nationalization, government officials having convinced them it would rescue the community from the industry's problems.[57] Also, the government had assured them that the Jeffrey Mine, the largest of its kind in the world, would have a leading role in the reorganization of the industry.

Nationalization was going to be the salvation of Asbestos. The new premier of Quebec had already proven himself to townspeople by rewriting many of the province's labour laws and passing Bill 45 in July 1977. This bill forbade the employment of strikebreakers during a legal strike, guaranteed the re-employment of striking workers once disputes were resolved, and implemented the mandatory contribution of union dues from all workers, unionized or not.[58] These reforms made Quebec a leader in North American labour legislation and were things the workers in Asbestos had wanted since 1949.

The PQ showed little concern for the multinational companies that owned many of the province's natural resources. Still believing the Jeffrey Mine was profitable, JM objected to government control of the industry. When this objection was leaked to the press in 1977, company president J.A. McKinney attempted to spin it in such a way as to avoid offending the provincial government in a time of industrial uncertainty. He wrote to Lévesque: "Our attitude from the beginning has been one of cooperation and not confrontation … We will continue to support your efforts to improve the economic well being of Quebec through betterment of the asbestos industry."[59]

The government passed Bill 70 in 1978 to form the Société nationale de l'amiante to promote the production and trade of the mineral. In turning the industry into a Crown corporation, the government spent $200 million buying the rights to the Thetford mines from the Asbestos Corporation and $50 million on plans for their expansion and promotion.[60] JM officials refused to sell the Jeffrey Mine, which they considered worth more than the province was offering. Unable to force a sale, the Quebec government became JM's leading Canadian competitor. The people of Asbestos were disaffected at remaining under the control of the American company, and they worried they would be left out of the government's plans to save the industry from collapse, especially when the first Fête de l'amiante was held in 1978 to promote and bring positive media attention to Thetford.

Community members attempted to boost the image of Asbestos by asking JM to repaint the exteriors of the factory buildings to beautify the town, but the company had a different strategy. In 1979, JM official J.R.M. Hutcheson wrote to Yves Bérubé, Quebec's environment minister, complaining that the company was paying 71 percent of its profits in taxes.[61]

Hutcheson said that the continuation of this tax burden would force the company to reconsider its future in Asbestos. The following year, in June 1980, when the Société nationale de l'amiante established a fixed price for asbestos, JM protested the policy and informed the government that it expected Jeffrey Mine shipments to decrease in the coming years because of the falling global demand for the mineral.[62]

The provincial government was beginning to realize that the industry was not as profitable or as stable as it seemed, and was no longer looking to expand its nationalization plans, so JM's protest was well timed. In September 1980, the company reduced the work week for 150 of its employees from six days to five;[63] then in January 1981, it laid off four hundred workers. Shift reductions and layoffs worried the people of Asbestos, who knew that the market was showing few signs of a rebound. The industry's decline in the early 1980s was very different from its troubles during the Great Depression, for it was rooted in something that would not change: the health effects of asbestos. Town council sought the advice of the Société nationale de l'amiante and formed a committee composed of the local union, the company, and the federal and provincial labour ministries to solve the unemployment problem in Asbestos.

JM owned and operated the Jeffrey Mine until 1983, but by 1981 it was no longer financially sustainable. Because of the tsunami of litigation the company faced in the United States, the continued collapse of the global industry, and the price-setting and taxation policies of the Quebec government, JM effectively gave up. The population of Asbestos had fallen from 10,254 in 1971 to 7,967 in 1981, and townspeople wanted to stop this exodus.[64] No longer viewing JM as a vital part of the community, council and unemployed workers held a series of meetings to address the crisis created by the collapse of the asbestos industry.

In a major policy shift, the Canadian Labour Congress (CLC) stopped attacking the industry's health effects on workers in order to help it survive.[65] When considering the best interests of its members, the union seemed to believe that jobs were more important than health. While it continued to advocate for occupational health and safety regulations to protect workers from industrial disease, the CLC no longer made the dangers of asbestos a major issue, stating instead that it could be extracted and processed safely if proper regulations were followed.

The people of Asbestos appreciated the union's support of their industry. Not knowing what the community would do if the market for asbestos collapsed, townspeople became comfortable with government protection, to the point of expecting it. The expectation of government aid reveals how dramatically the once fiercely independent townspeople changed to adapt to the realities of a collapsing industry. Council used government money to create new jobs for its citizens, generating 72 temporary positions for the summer and then an additional 114.[66] These efforts were not enough to sustain the failing community. In March, the Unemployment Committee of Asbestos requested that the local outdoor skating rink remain open as long as weather allowed and asked for the donation of a ping-pong table in order to give unemployed Jeffrey Mine workers something to do.[67] Asbestos had become a place where people drifted from activity to activity with no real purpose and no real connection to the Jeffrey Mine.

Over the years, the people of Asbestos had negotiated a balance between the interests of the workers, the company, and council, but when JM began to opt out, equilibrium was lost. Council funded activities for its unemployed citizens, but it did not succeed in generating permanent jobs. The Jeffrey Mine defined Asbestos and was the community's reason to exist. Aside from providing temporary summer jobs and activities, the town could do little to help its citizens.

Representatives from the provincial and the federal governments thought they could do more to support Asbestos than the community's town council. Town officials met with PQ cabinet minister Yves Duhaime in March 1982 to discuss provincial aid for the community. Duhaime had just returned from a European trip to evaluate the global market for asbestos, and he believed the industry would soon rebound. In June 1982, the Department of National Defence contacted town council to extend its business agreement for another five years. This meant that Jeffrey Mine fibre would continue to be used in military equipment despite growing health concerns. The federal government also showed its support at Montreal's 1982 World Symposium on Asbestos when the industry minister, Herb Grey, spoke out against the European countries that had banned asbestos. Grey actively sought out new markets for the Canadian mineral in developing nations.[68] He declared that nine out of ten Canadian provinces supported the continuation of the industry, believing that the health risks were manageable. He did not say where this statistic came from.

Reinvention possibilities were limited for a town named Asbestos, but while its population was not large and the revenue from its industry dwindled each year, the community refused to accept collapse. International markets were rapidly closing their doors to asbestos products, and there was no sign the public's negative opinion of the mineral would change. The landscape of the Eastern Townships was scarred by a century of mining, and Asbestos and Thetford were too far away from Montreal and

Quebec City to be viable for smaller-scale industrial development: without asbestos they would die. Refusing to believe this, the Quebec government chose to sustain the asbestos industry and its collapsed communities financially and politically to avoid having to address the problem of entire towns of unemployed workers.

Although JM did not see a future in Asbestos, it asked the Canadian government for $35 million to support the industry. An earlier Récupération Régionale Richmond-Wolfe project had only created nine new jobs in the region,[69] so chances were good that the government would grant JM this funding, given that mining asbestos was the only way the community could survive. At the start of February 1983, JM told town council that the company was optimistic about the Jeffrey Mine's future.[70] The company's optimism was contagious, and townspeople expressed theirs by organizing community activities to keep spirits up while waiting to be taken back to work at the Jeffrey Mine. Their hope was short-lived. A week later, JM revoked its request for money from the federal government. The company would not rehire any of its laid-off workers, and in June 1983 it left Asbestos after selling the Jeffrey Mine to a handful of former JM executives. The town now had to solve its problems alone.

In the spring of 1983, council allocated half a million dollars to attract new industry to Asbestos. It also partnered with the federal employment and immigration minister, Lloyd Axworthy, and the Société nationale de l'amiante to create three hundred new jobs, and it received federal funds for further industrial development.[71] Despite these efforts, no major industry came to the town. Projects and government subsidies continued to pour into Asbestos, and for a time there were hopes the community would become a regional centre for a variety of educational and health services. Both hope and effort were in vain, and the community entered a period of prolonged uncertainty and decline.

Surviving Collapse:
Asbestos Post-1983

WHAT'S IN A NAME? Asbestos by any other name would still have the massive mine at the centre of the community, its economy, and its history. Federal and provincial government subsidies sustained the Jeffrey Mine – and the people of Asbestos – until 2012, when operations were finally halted for good. From 1983 to 2012, the people of Asbestos did everything in their power to ensure the continuation of the industry. Throughout this book, we have repeatedly seen this community's resilience and ability to survive. Now it enters a new phase. How does a long-established resource community survive market collapse? How does it reconcile the historical and local understanding of its resource with new understandings of the harms it inflicted and continues to inflict today? How does one go to sleep at night next to a 2 kilometre opencast asbestos mine? These are all difficult questions the people of Asbestos have had to answer since 1983 while dealing with their own economic instability and health concerns.

In June 2010, the Canadian Cancer Society wrote to the Quebec government urging it to stop supporting the industry because asbestos continues to cause the deaths of around 90,000 people annually all over the world.[1] The people of Asbestos reacted immediately and fiercely to this perceived attack and cancelled the town's annual Relay for Life, for which they had raised almost $350,000 for cancer research in the previous four years. André Beaulieu, a representative from the Canadian Cancer Society, attributed townspeople's reaction to local economic concerns, but Mayor Hughes Grimard challenged Beaulieu's assumption, explaining that "we want to work with our partners and not with our detractors … It's our past, it's our history, therefore the population is united in support of the mining industry."[2] The community, although battered by recent realities, remains strongly committed to the collapsed industry. The cancers the people of Asbestos are suffering from are fast acting, painful, and often incurable, yet by diminishing the mineral's negative health effects on their own bodies, Jeffrey Mine workers have contributed to the perpetuation of the deadly cycle of work and disease around the world, most recently in those developing countries to which Canada sold the mineral until 2012.

THE ARGUMENT IN SUMMARY

The preceding pages have explored the local-global tensions created by environmental change and contamination in a resource community. They have also explored the many ways that townspeople defined survival, and fought for it, during the rise and fall of the industry. JM played a leading role in the history of the global asbestos trade, but so too did the environment itself and the residents of Asbestos. These people were not the industry's only miners, and they were not its only French Canadian workers; that said, the ways the community interpreted its local role in the global industry complicate and challenge the international literature on the asbestos industry. Closely examined, the story of Asbestos involves deceitful international corporations prioritizing profits over human life, but it also highlights the complex interactions between people and their local environment.

The history of Asbestos is what it is because of a geological quirk. The massive circular mineral deposit in the centre of the community was as unusual as it was profitable, and was an ideal source for companies that wanted large amounts of raw asbestos. Furthermore, the community itself was ideal, for it was close enough to the major port cities of Montreal, Quebec City, and Portland, Maine, not to mention the St Lawrence Seaway, that companies could easily ship asbestos all over the world. As connected as this made Asbestos to the rest of the world, the community remained isolated from major medical discoveries and labour movements happening elsewhere, largely because of language and culture. That most Jeffrey Mine employees were French Canadian, that they belonged to a Quebec-based union rooted in the principles of the Catholic Church, and that they lived in a province with a legal system that limited the action they could take against JM for occupational health compensation, further isolated the community from global industrial trends.

Before the large-scale extraction of asbestos, the landscape around the town was part of the rolling Appalachian Mountains, and asbestos-related disease did not kill 90,000 people every year. Then society's increasing demand for the comfort and convenience that materials like asbestos offered to households, industries, and transportation companies in the nineteenth and twentieth centuries radically altered the land and the ways it affected human health. The Jeffrey Mine was not the only part of the global asbestos industry, but its workers contributed significantly to the proliferation of the mineral around the world.

JM did not willingly give up its place as a leader in the global asbestos industry; rather, it was forced to do so by a collapsing market and by rising lawsuits launched against the company by its American workers. Similarly, the people of Asbestos did not willingly give up their role as a main supplier to the global industry; rather, they were forced to do so by increased domestic and international concerns about the mineral and by an effective anti-asbestos lobbying campaign that eventually, in 2012, convinced the Quebec government to withhold its financial and political support.³ Since 1983, JM has redefined itself as a producer of non-asbestos-containing building supplies. The rebranding of the town of Asbestos has not been so easy, for the physical reality of the Jeffrey Mine prevents the local population and potential investors from seeing beyond the industry.

By working the Jeffrey Mine and sacrificing local land to its development, townspeople contributed a considerable percentage of the global supply of the mineral. Furthermore, by unknowingly acting as test mice in a giant living laboratory, they supplied JM with crucial knowledge of asbestos-related disease – knowledge that proved beyond doubt that the Canadian mineral was deadly. The company kept this information from those suffering asbestos-linked diseases, as well as from the general public; indeed, it was JM's insistence that Jeffrey Mine workers were healthy and that Canadian chrysotile was inert that kept the Quebec industry alive for so long. To keep the Jeffrey Mine open after 1983, townspeople adopted JM's mantra that they were not sick and that the mineral was safe. This false information led directly to the proliferation of asbestos throughout the developing world, negatively affecting workers and other citizens who did not have access to the literature about the deadly mineral's risks, or to dust elimination technologies. Asbestos-related disease rates continue to rise in these countries, and Jeffrey Mine workers contributed to this reality. The community and the industry's supporters wielded astonishing power in Canadian politics, and together they convinced government officials to use Canada's positive international image to block the strict global regulation of chrysotile asbestos. This occurred at the provincial *and* federal levels of government for almost thirty years and gave the people of Asbestos the false impression that their industry – and perhaps their community – could survive.

RISK AND SOCIETY

This study has also shown how the history of asbestos played out at a local level. The mineral was put to so many domestic and industrial uses because manufacturers and consumers trusted that it was safe and that it would protect them from other hazards, such as fire. The community at the heart of this study boomed during this "Golden Age of Asbestos." However, much like what happened with the tobacco industry, companies could not hide the negative health effects of the mineral forever, and when the day came, the economy of Asbestos began to crumble. As awareness grew of the fibre's risks, large-scale anti-asbestos campaigns throughout the Western world – including in Canada – succeeded in having the mineral taken out of homes, schools, hospitals, and other public spaces.

These pages have shown that society's handling of the risks asbestos posed was not a simple black-and-white case of cause and effect, discovery and renunciation. British workers were dying of asbestos-related disease by the start of the twentieth century. The first documented case of an American Johns-Manville employee becoming ill because of the mineral was in the 1920s. Jeffrey Mine workers launched a long, industry-wide strike in 1949 because of the sudden, widespread awareness of the negative effects of asbestos on human health. This was all part of the public record, and, especially in the case of the 1949 strike, part of the political and medical dialogue of the day. But it was not until Western society came to understand the risks asbestos posed to the general public, rather than simply to the working class, that lobby groups really began to launch effective campaigns against the mineral. Does society expect miners and other members of the working class, including those in developing countries, to get sick? Does society tolerate these environmental and industrial hazards as long as the white middle and upper classes are not affected? The history of Asbestos suggests this could indeed be the case.

The collapse of Asbestos was unlike that of other mining communities such as Cobalt, Ontario, and St. Clair, Pennsylvania, because the local mineral deposits were not exhausted. It was also different from the bust of the uranium towns of the American West, which survive to this day by marketing their communities to tourists seeking 1950s nostalgia.[4] Furthermore, Jeffrey Mine employees never romanticized their labour like Cape Breton coal miners, who sing in the world-renowned Men of the Deeps choir and put a positive, friendly image on another deadly industry – an image that allowed them to lobby successfully for new coal mines as recently as May 2010.[5] Instead, the collapse of the asbestos industry and the town of Asbestos was caused solely by the dangers the mineral posed to human health, and the community has been left with a massive opencast mine containing a fibre that has the potential to harm an unknown number of people.

ENVIRONMENT AND IDENTITY

This book has aimed to show how changing international perceptions of asbestos affected its namesake town of Asbestos. As demand for the mineral grew, so did local pride in land and labour: Jeffrey Mine workers believed they were helping make the world a safer place. The West's gradual rejection of asbestos because of its negative effects on human health created great confusion for the community. Workers were not doing anything differently from what generations of Jeffrey Mine employees had done, but the fruits of their labours were generating a reaction much different from that they had once received. They were suddenly forced to think about what their commitment to the industry said about them and their future. The impact the terminal decline of the asbestos industry had on the local identity was considerable, and still is. The years since 1983 have been marked by the steady but also sweeping local-global reorientation of Asbestos, and the community has shrunk in size, hovering between 6,000 to 7,000 citizens since 2001. Schools are boarded up, houses are for sale, and the town's political, economic, and societal foundations have been profoundly shaken by the industry's collapse.

This study has examined the environmental change, contamination, and survival of one resource community. As mentioned in the Introduction, the insistence of G. Claude Théroux of the Société d'Histoire d'Asbestos that we must understand asbestos the mineral in order to understand Asbestos the place was the foundation of this analysis. Everything in the community's history occurred in the extreme: land exploitation, profits, labour disputes, disease, global renown, and industrial collapse. But at the same time, if not for the extremes of the land, and the mineral found deep within it, the town of Asbestos would not exist. Every decision made by the working class, the town councillors, and JM officials was done with consideration of the land and how it would affect the future of the industry and the community that relied on it. Over their history, the people of Asbestos developed a sense of ownership of the Jeffrey Mine and a balanced system of land use, which they never hesitated to defend. The local population also developed a sense of trust in the land, and it was difficult for them to accept that it was dangerous: after all, this was their home.

The remarkable history of identity in Asbestos was rooted in a local understanding of the environment, health, and community. Agricultural land has been important in much of Quebec's past; the history of Asbestos has shown us how people can also have complex relationships with an industrialized landscape. This book should encourage us to question our assumptions about how people and the natural environment relate to each other, and to reconsider how residents of resource communities understand and manage risk. This would give us a more holistic understanding of commodity flows, environmental health, and the interconnectedness of local-global politics. It would also help us create solutions to the problems facing collapsed resource communities by specifically addressing the local attachment to the natural environment those communities live and labour in, and to the global trade networks they once supplied.

This study of a single community has also been a study of massive environmental change, controversial health and safety issues, and clashes between local and international responsibilities. The experiences the community, the province, and the nation have gained through the history of Asbestos can lead to a re-evaluation of how Canada processes and markets its natural resources today. Many parallels can be drawn between Asbestos and the Athabasca Oil Sands, given that millions rely on the oil found in communities like Fort McMurray, just as people once relied on the asbestos found in the Jeffrey Mine. Huge international corporations are radically changing Alberta's environment because of the global demand for oil, despite the fact that international organizations are working towards reducing the use of petroleum because of its negative effects on the environment and human health.

The situation unfolding in places like Fort McMurray mirrors what happened in Asbestos when the public became aware of the mineral's health risks. Just like asbestos was for Quebec, oil is an important driver of wealth and employment in Alberta, as well as a fundamental part of the local identity and economy. If a reliable, more environmentally sustainable replacement for oil comes to market, communities like Fort McMurray could face terminal decline, just like Asbestos did. The only thing left would be an industrialized environment that is no longer viable, populated by people who no longer have stable employment opportunities. Canada has a long history as a resource colony, extracting raw materials from the land and shipping them around the world.[6] Resource industries continue to fuel the economy, and this study has shown that Canadian society needs to re-evaluate how it manages its environmental and economic ambitions, which thus far are fairly unchecked.

There is an intimacy between life and labour in resource communities. The way land, people, and politics interacted in Asbestos illustrates how humans form connections with the natural world. In Asbestos, the land is more than dangerous, the people are more than statistics, and the community is not something that history just happened to. This was and is a living, breathing, working society. By remembering how the land, the people, and the community historically depended on each other for existence, we can draw broader conclusions about the ways in which nature and culture interact. The Jeffrey Mine remains a massive presence in the community, and asbestos-related disease continues to affect local residents, as well as tens of thousands of people around the world. The history of environmental change, contamination, and survival in Asbestos is slowly coming to an end but continues to have significant local and global effects. The Jeffrey Mine is so large and so central to the town that it cannot be covered up or ignored. Asbestos cannot be reinvented easily. Although the industry has collapsed, and in many ways so has the town, the people of Asbestos remain committed to their past, waiting for a new creation story.

Notes

FOREWORD

1 Louise Penny, *The Long Way Home* (London: Little, Brown, 2014). Quotations in this paragraph from chapters 1 and 2.
2 Penny, *Long Way Home*, chapter 35.
3 Penny, *Long Way Home*, quotations from chapter 36.
4 In her acknowledgments, Penny recognizes the influence of Marilynne Robinson's "remarkable" book *Gilead* (Farrar, Strauss and Giroux, 2004) as well as the old spiritual "Balm in Gilead," Joseph Conrad's *Heart of Darkness*, and Homer's *Odyssey*. Penny, *Long Way Home*.
5 Brett L. Walker, *Toxic Archipelago: A History of Industrial Disease in Japan* (Seattle/London: University of Washington Press, 2010).
6 Rachel Carson, *Silent Spring* (New York: Houghton Mifflin, 1962).
7 John Keats, "La Belle Dame sans Merci," (1820); the relevant lines are: "The sedge is wither'd from the lake, And no birds sing." Quotes in the remainder of this paragraph are from Rachel Carson, "A Fable for Tomorrow," in *Silent Spring*, 1-3.
8 Rob Nixon, *Slow Violence and the Environmentalism of the Poor* (Cambridge, MA: Harvard University Press, 2011). Quote from Rob Nixon, "Slow Violence," *The Chronicle of Higher Education*, 26 June 2011. For discussion of a parallel case, in the making of the film *The Day after Tomorrow* about a sudden climate shift, "modelled" after that in the Younger Dryas, see Franz Mauelshagen, "Climate Catastrophism: The History of the Future of Climate Change," in *Historical Disasters in Context: Science, Religion, and Politics*, ed. A. Janku, F. Mauelshagen, and G. Schenk (London/New York: Routledge, 2012), 261-82, who quotes the film's director Roland Emmerich in defence of this approach: "Of course we dramatized the process. You cannot make a film which dabbles on over three or four years."
9 Nixon, *Slow Violence*, 9.
10 Linda Lear, *Rachel Carson: Witness for Nature* (New York: Henry Holt and Company, 1997); Eliza Griswold, "How 'Silent Spring' Ignited the Environmental Movement," *New York*

Times Magazine, 21 September 2012. Available at: http://mobile.nytimes.com/2012/09/23/ magazine/how-silent-spring-ignited-the-environmental-movement.html?pagewanted= all&_r=0.

11 H. Patricia Hynes, *The Recurring Silent Spring* (New York: Pergamon Press, 1989), 3.

12 Graeme Wynn, "The Power of Words and the Tides of History: Reflections on *Man and Nature* and *Silent Spring*," in *Geographies of Knowledge and Power (Knowledge and Space)*, ed. Peter Meusburger, Derek Gregory, and Laura Suarsana (Springer Netherlands, forthcoming 2015), Knowledge and Space Series No. 7.

13 Nixon, *Slow Violence*, 40.

14 Frantz Fanon, *The Wretched of the Earth*, translated by Constance Farrington (New York: Grove Weidenfeld, 1963), 38.

15 Naomi Oreskes and Erik M. Conway, *Merchants of Doubt* (New York: Bloomsbury, 2010).

16 The million-fibrils-an-inch estimate comes from Steven Schwarze, "Silences and Possibilities of Asbestos Activism: Stories from Libby," in *Environmental Justice and Environmentalism: The Social Justice Challenge to The Environmental Movement*, ed. Ronald D. Sandler and Phaedra C. Pezzullo (Cambridge MA: MIT Press, 2007), 165-87. This short account offers a useful complement to *A Town Called Asbestos* especially on points in the mid-latter part of this paragraph. For fuller commentaries, see A. Peacock, *Libby, Montana: Asbestos and the Deadly Silence of an American Corporation* (Boulder, CO: Johnson Books, 2003), and A. Schneider and D. McCumber, *An Air that Kills: How the Asbestos Poisoning of Libby, Montana Uncovered a National Scandal* (New York: Putnam, 2004). Also *Libby, Montana: A Film by Drury Gunn Carr and Doug Hawes-Davis*. Summary and guide available at: http://pov-tc.pbs.org/pov/downloads/2007/pov-libbymontana-discussion-guide-color.pdf. The Libby story was "broken" by A. Schneider, "Uncivil Action: A Town Left to Die," *Seattle Post-Intelligencer*, November 18, 1999.

17 Tavia Grant, "Asbestos Revealed as Canada's Top Cause of Workplace Death," *The Globe and Mail Report on Business,* December 15, 2014. Available at: http://www.theglobe andmail.com/report-on-business/asbestos-is-canadas-top-source-of-workplace-death/article 22081291/. See also, Tavia Grant, "No Safe Use: Canada's Embrace of the 'Miracle Mineral' has Seeded an Epidemic of Cancers – Yet Many Canadians Are Still Exposed to Asbestos Every Day." A seven-part series with video, available online (nd) at: http://www.the globeandmail.com/report-on-business/no-safe-use-as-the-top-workplace-killer-asbestos -leaves-a-deadly-legacy/article19151351/. For a background report on the series, see Tavia Grant, "Explore the Data and Details behind *The Globe's* Project on the Dangers of Asbestos," *The Globe and Mail*, June 16, 2014. Available at: http://www.theglobeandmail. com/report-on-business/explore-the-data-and-details-behind-the-globes-project-on-the -dangers-of-asbestos/article19154101/#dashboard/follows/. Some estimates from the early 2000s place the annual number of deaths from asbestos-related cancers worldwide at 100,000 to 140,000.

18 Marlene Harris, "Review of *The Long Way Home*," August 22nd, 2014, Reading Reality Blog. Available at: http://www.readingreality.net/2014/08/review-the-long-way-home-by -louise-penny/.

19 Charles Isherwood, "Trailing an Artist Who Lost His Way," *New York Times*, August 28, 2014. Available at: http://www.nytimes.com/2014/08/29/books/louise-pennys-the-long -way-home.html?_r=0.

20 Said quoted in Nixon, "Slow Violence," 6.

Introduction

1   Interview with G. Claude Théroux, Société d'Histoire d'Asbestos, December 2007.
2   The term "serpentine" designates a "specific mineral species that was hydrated and contained magnesium and silica … [they are] massive, lamellar, columnar, or fibrous." "Amphibole" refers to a different mineral group, many of which resemble sharp needles under a microscope, and can "occur as chunky, acicular, or equant crystals, as well as in fibrous form." H. Catherine W. Skinner, Malcolm Ross, and Clifford Frondel, *Asbestos and Other Fibrous Minerals* (Oxford: Oxford University Press, 1988), 196, 33.
3   Maines, *Asbestos and Fire*, 27–28; Tweedale, *Magic Mineral to Killer Dust*, 2.
4   Cornelis Klein, "Rocks, Minerals, and a Dusty World," in *Reviews in Mineralogy: Health Effects of Mineral Dusts*, ed. Brooke T. Mossman and George D. Guthrie Jr. (Chelsea: Mineralogical Society of America, 1993), 17.
5   Tweedale, *Magic Mineral to Killer Dust*, 2.
6   David Robertson, *Hard as the Rock Itself: Place and Identity in the American Mining Town*, Boulder: University of Colorado Press, 2010, 3.
7   Patricia A. McAnany and Norman Yoffee, eds., "Why We Question Collapse and Study Human Resilience, Ecological Vulnerability, and the Aftermath of Empire," in *Questioning Collapse: Human Resilience, Ecological Vulnerability, and the Aftermath of Empire* (Cambridge: Cambridge University Press, 2009), 5-6.
8   Anthony C. Gatrell and Susan J. Elliott, *Geographies of Health: An Introduction*, 2nd ed. (Malden: Wiley-Blackwell, 2009), 44. See also William M. Gesler and Robin A. Kearns, *Culture/Place/Health* (New York: Routledge, 2002); and Florence M. Margai, *Environmental Health Hazards and Social Justice: Geographical Perspectives on Race and Class Disparities* (London: Earthscan, 2010).
9   Richard White, "'Are You an Environmentalist or Do You Work for a Living?': Work and Nature," in *Uncommon Ground: Toward Reinventing Nature*, ed. William Cronon (New York: W.W. Norton, 1995), 172; White, *The Organic Machine*, 113.
10 Rajala, *Clearcutting the Pacific Rainforest*, 30.
11 See, for example, Logan Hovis and Jeremy Mouat, "Miners, Engineers, and the Transformation of Work in the Western Mining Industry, 1889–1930," *Technology and Culture* 37, 3 (July 1996): 429-56; Piper, *The Industrial Transformation of Subarctic Canada*; and David A. Wolff, *Industrializing the Rockies: Growth, Competition, and Turmoil in the Coalfields of Colorado and Wyoming, 1868–1914* (Boulder: University Press of Colorado, 2003).
12 David Cantor, "The Diseased Body," in *Medicine in the Twentieth Century*, ed. Roger Cooter and John Pickstone, (London: Taylor and Francis, 2000), 347. For more studies on occupational health and industrial medicine that attempt to get away from this historiographical trend, see Judkins, *We Offer Ourselves as Evidence*.
13 See, for example, Braun and Truan, "An Epidemiological Study"; and John Corbett McDonald, McGill University, "Report," 1972, QAMA, 4–9.
14 See, for example, Jean Dubois, *The White Plague: Tuberculosis, Man and Society* (New Brunswick: Rutgers University Press, 1987); Nadja Durbach, "'They Might as Well Brand Us': Working-Class Resistance to Compulsory Vaccination in Victorian England," *Social History of Medicine* 13, 1 (2000): 45–63; and Sheila M. Rothman, *Living in the Shadow of Death: Tuberculosis and the Social Experience of Illness in American History* (Baltimore: Johns Hopkins University Press, 1995).

15 Douglas, *Risk and Blame*, 30; and Beck, *Risk Society*, 24.
16 Parr, *Sensing Changes*, 8 (emphasis hers).
17 See, for example, Andrews, *Killing for Coal*; Buckly, *Danger, Death, and Disaster*.
18 Historical perspectives on the Quiet Revolution vary. See, for example, Behiels, *Prelude to Quebec's Quiet Revolution*; Linteau et al., *Quebec: A History, 1867–1929*; McRoberts, *Quebec*; and Vallières, *White Niggers of America*.
19 Trudeau, "Introduction," *The Asbestos Strike*, 67.
20 The industry collapsed in the early 1980s, but as recent as 2010, the federal government gave pro-asbestos lobby groups a quarter of a million dollars, promoted the mineral in international markets, and prevented the UN from banning trading of the mineral. The Quebec government also supports the industry, and in June 2010 it backed a $58 million bank loan to further develop the Jeffrey Mine and sustain the dwindling local workforce for at least twenty-five more years. See "Asbestos Mine Workers to Build Reserve Fund," *CBC News*, June 14, 2010, http://www.cbc.ca/news/canada/montreal/asbestos-mine -workers-to-build-reserve-fund-1.911473; and Kathleen Ruff, "Deathbed Reprieve for Killer Industry?" *Toronto Star*, June 6, 2010.
21 This is certainly not the first study that focuses on the corporate crime of companies like Johns-Manville. JM and other asbestos manufacturing companies like Britain's Turner & Newall had a long history of suppressing medical knowledge and gaining government allies to ensure industry profits while knowingly putting workers and community members at environmental and occupational risk. Please see Tweedale, *Magic Mineral to Killer Dust*; McCulloch and Tweedale, *Defending the Indefensible*; Egilman, Fehnel, and Bohme, "Exposing the 'Myth' of ABC"; Brodeur, *Expendable Americans*; and Markowitz and Rosner, *Deceit and Denial*.
22 See for example, Christopher C. Sellers, *Hazards of the Job: From Industrial Disease to Environmental Health Science* (Chapel Hill: University of North Carolina Press, 1997).

Chapter 1: Creation Stories

1 Ryan, "Caledonides"; Rothery, "Obduction"; O'Hanley, "The Origin of the Chrysotile Asbestos Veins," 8.
2 Vallières, *Des Mines et des Hommes*, 63.
3 Murray, "Report of Alexander Murray, Esq.," 388. "Asbestus" was an alternative spelling of "asbestos" at this time.
4 Vallières, *Des Mines et des Hommes*, 95.
5 "Geological Survey of Canada: Report for the Year 1919," 5A.
6 Armstrong, "Le Développement des Droits Miniers au Québec," 581.
7 Lampron, Cantin, and Grimard, *Asbestos*, 37.
8 Cirkel, *Asbestos*, 31.
9 Robert Armstrong, "The Quebec Asbestos Industry: Technological Change, 1878–1929," in Cameron, ed., *Explorations in Canadian Economic History*, 191.
10 Obalski, *Mines and Minerals*, 97.
11 Ostry, *Change and Continuity*, 167; and Michael Bliss, "Growth, Progress, and the Quest for Salvation: Confessions of a Medical Historian," in Heaman, Li, and McKellar, eds., *Essays in Honour of Michael Bliss*.
12 MacDermot, *History of the CMA, 1867–1921*, vol. 1, 138; and Grenier, *100 Ans de Médicine*, 9.

13 Cirkel, *Asbestos,* 30.

14 Lampron, Cantin, and Grimard, *Asbestos,* 63.

15 "Geological Survey of Canada: Report for the Year 1886," 30A.

16 Ibid., 50A.

17 Ibid., 50A.

18 Ibid., 2A.

19 Obalski, *Mines and Minerals,* 107–8, 159.

20 "Geological Survey of Canada: Report for the Year 1886," 31A.

21 Obalski, *Mines and Minerals,* 91.

22 *Canadian Mining and Mechanical Review,* vol. 9 (February 1890), 16. This monograph employs a variety of "tons" throughout, but makes clear which unit is being employed according to the source material. Most weight measurements are given in the English, or long, ton, which is 2,240 lbs. and is the measurement most of my sources employ. So unless noted, that is the weight I am referring to. The American or short ton, which is 2,000 lbs., is also used on occasion, but noted each time. The metric tonne, 2,204.6 lbs., is rarely used in my sources, but when it is, I use it and note it.

23 Obalski, *Mines and Minerals,* 91.

24 Armstrong, "Le Développement des Droits Miniers au Québec," 585.

25 Obalski, *Mines and Minerals,* 108.

26 Robert H. Jones, *Asbestos and Asbestic: Their Properties, Occurrence, and Use* (London: Crosby Lockwood and Son, 1897): 171.

27 Geological Survey of Canada: Report for the Year 1887, 112K.

28 Obalski, *Mines and Minerals,* 95.

29 *Canadian Mining and Mechanical Review,* 10, 1 (January 1891): 210.

30 "A Visit to the Shipton Mines," *Richmond Guardian,* July 9, 1892, 1.

31 Robert H. Jones, "Asbestos and Asbestic," 187.

32 *Canadian Mining and Mechanical Review,* 11 (1892): 32, 149.

33 *Canadian Mining and Mechanical Review,* 10, 1 (1891): 204.

34 "Quebec Tax on Mining," *Canadian Mining and Mechanical Review,* 10, 2 (1891): 1.

35 *Canadian Mining Review,* vol. 13 (1894): 84.

36 Jones, "Asbestos and Asbestic," p. 187.

37 Jones, *Asbestos and Asbestic,* 175.

38 *Canadian Mining Review* (October 1896): 218.

39 *Canadian Mining Review,* vol. 14 (1895): 182.

40 Linteau et al., *Quebec: A History,* 305.

41 Jones, *Asbestos and Asbestic,* 170.

42 Boas, "Composition of Matter for Wall-Plaster," 2.

43 Ibid., 1.

44 *Canadian Mining Review* (November 1897): 324.

45 Jones, *Asbestos and Asbestic,* 183–84.

46 Obalski wrote reports in both French and English. Obalski, *Province de Québec,* 35.

47 While the company remained the H.W. Johns-Manville Co. until 1930, I will hereafter refer to it as Johns-Manville and JM to ensure consistency, as the name change did not mark any significant changes in corporate structure.

48 *Canadian Mining Review,* vol. 12 (January 1893): 4.

49 Cirkel, *Asbestos,* 32.

50 Cirkel, *Asbestos,* 23, 102.

51 "Village d'Asbestos un centre prospere qui deviendra la Ville d'Asbestos et aussi, a ciel ouvert, la plus grande mine d'amiante au monde." English translation by author, *L'Asbestos*, March 4, 1949, 1, March 11, 1949, 1, and March 18, 1949, 1.
52 Ibid., 192.
53 Ibid., 191.
54 *Sherbrooke Daily Record*, May 27, 1909, 1.
55 Vallières, *Des Mines et des Hommes*, 55.
56 *Canadian Mining Journal*, June 15, 1909, 362.
57 Vallières, *Des Mines et des Hommes*, 129; and *Sherbrooke La Tribune*, September 3, 1912, 7.
58 *Annuaire Statistique de Québec*, 286.
59 *Annuaire Statistique de Québec*, 286.
60 *L'Asbestos*, April 29, 1949, 1.
61 *Canadian Mining Journal*, November 1, 1914, 712.
62 W.C. Clarke Fonds, Eastern Townships Research Centre, photo C14.
63 Lampron, Cantin, and Grimard, *Asbestos*, 49; Armstrong, "The Quebec Asbestos Industry," 204.
64 *Canadian Mining Journal*, March 1, 1918, 90.

Chapter 2: Land with a Future, Not a Past, 1918-49

1 "How to Sell Asbestos, Canada," *Gruen Transfer*, http://www.abc.net.au/tv/gruentransfer. For access to the commercial in Canada, see https://www.youtube.com/watch?v=KIpxelbkIoI.
2 Vallières, *Des Mines et des Hommes*, 105.
3 W.G. Clarke. W.G. Clarke Fonds, Eastern Townships Research Centre.
4 *Procès-verbal*, La ville d'Asbestos, May 23, 1918, 143.
5 *Procès-verbal*, La ville d'Asbestos, June 2, 1918, 146.
6 Summers, *Asbestos and the Asbestos Industry*, 8.
7 *Canadian Mining Journal*, December 24, 1919, 966.
8 Summers, *Asbestos and the Asbestos Industry*, 1–2.
9 *Canadian Mining Journal*. December 31, 1920, 1079, and January 7, 1920, 4.
10 *Canadian Mining Journal*. July 22, 1921, 576.
11 *Procès-verbal*, La ville d'Asbestos, March 14, 1923, 407.
12 Vallières, *Des Mines et des Hommes*, 165.
13 "Modernization of the Asbestos Mines," *Canadian Mining Journal*, August 5, 1921, 618.
14 Norman A. Fisher, "The Quebec Asbestos Industry," *Canadian Mining Journal*, August 17, 1923, 649.
15 "si essentiel à la vie et l'intérêt de la communauté locale," *Procès-verbal*, La ville d'Asbestos, November 13, 1923, 447. English translation by author.
16 Lampron, Cantin, and Grimard, *Asbestos*, 117.
17 "The Canadian Johns-Manville Co. Ltd. Work on a Large Scale," *Canadian Mining Journal*, January 4, 1924, 30.
18 *Canadian Mining Journal*, April 18, 1924, 374.
19 *Procès-verbal*, La ville d'Asbestos, April 27, 1927, 137.
20 Lampron, Cantin, and Grimard, *Asbestos*, 140.
21 *Procès-verbal*, La ville d'Asbestos, March 4, 1926, 68–69.
22 "Commence à grignoter le village," *Le Citoyen*, December 28, 1974, 70. English translation by author.

23 *Le Citoyen,* December 28, 1974, 42. This phrase was also used in a 1967 article on the expansion of the Jeffrey Mine: Ross, "Encroachment of the Jeffrey Mine."

24 *Asbestos: Its Sources,* 17.

25 Gillies, "The Asbestos Industry," 40.

26 "Apporte la presque totalité des revenues d'Asbestos," *L'Asbestos,* August 26, 1949, 1. English translation by author.

27 *Le Citoyen,* December 28, 1974, 70.

28 *Procès-verbal,* La ville d'Asbestos, January 11, 1932, 429, and June 1, 1932, 470.

29 McCulloch and Tweedale, *Defending the Indefensible,* 26.

30 Oliver Bowles and B.H. Stoddard, "Asbestos," in *Minerals Yearbook 1934,* ed. O.E. Kiessling (Washington: US GPO, 1934), 1014.

31 Oliver Bowles and M.A. Cornthwaite, "Asbestos," *Minerals Yearbook 1937,* ed. Herbert H. Hughes (Washington: US GPO, 1937), 1368.

32 *Canadian Mining Journal,* February 1938, 65.

33 Bowles and Cornthwaite, "Asbestos," 1363.

34 *Johns-Manville News Pictorial,* December 1938, 4.

35 *Procès-verbal,* La ville d'Asbestos, September 30, 1938, 158.

36 Ross, "Encroachment of the Jeffrey Mine," 529.

37 *Procès-verbal,* La ville d'Asbestos, January 3, 1939, 182; *Procès-verbal,* La ville d'Asbestos, April 3, 1939, 210.

38 R.C. Rowe, "Mining and Milling Operations of the Canadian Johns-Manville Company Ltd. at Asbestos, PQ," *Canadian Mining Journal,* April 1939, 185.

39 Ibid., 190.

40 Ibid., 194.

41 Ibid., 194.

42 For more on this connection, see Andrews, *Killing for Coal;* and White, *The Organic Machine.*

43 Oliver Bowles and K.G. Warner, "Asbestos," *Minerals Yearbook 1939,* ed. Herbert Hughes (Washington: US GPO, 1939), 1309.

44 McCulloch and Tweedale, *Defending the Indefensible,* 28.

45 Elizabeth W. Gillies, "The Asbestos Industry Since 1929 with Special Reference to Canada," MA thesis, McGill University, 1941, 8.

46 *Procès-verbal,* La ville d'Asbestos, May 6, 1942, 495.

47 *Procès-verbal,* La ville d'Asbestos, June 22, 1942, 3 and 5, and February 8, 1943, 36.

48 McCulloch and Tweedale, *Defending the Indefensible,* 28.

49 *Procès-verbal,* La ville d'Asbestos, June 16, 1943, 50, and July 7, 1943, 52.

50 Oliver Bowles and F.M. Barsigian, "Asbestos," *Minerals Yearbook 1943,* ed. E.W. Pehrson and C.E. Needham (Washington: US GPO, 1943), 1431.

51 *Procès-verbal,* La ville d'Asbestos, August 9, 1944, 8.

52 This figure refers to American tons, which are 2,000 lbs. One of these new products was asbestos sheeting, invented in Britain, which was able to withstand extremely high temperature and pressure and was suitable for both fighter jets and commercial airlines. Oliver Bowles and Dorothy I. Marsh, "Asbestos," *Minerals Yearbook 1944,* ed. E.W. Pehrson and C.E. Needham (Washington: United States Printing Office, 1944), 1478.

53 G.W. Josephson and Dorothy I. Marsh, "Asbestos," *Minerals Yearbook 1946,* ed. E.W. Pehrson and Allen F. Matthews (Washington: US GPO, 1946), 150.

54 "à défendre les intérêts de la Ville d'Asbestos," *Procès-verbal,* La ville d'Asbestos, November 6, 1946, 199. English translation by author.

55 *Procès-verbal*, La ville d'Asbestos, November 6, 1946, 199.
56 "Règlement No. 240," *Procès-verbal*, La ville d'Asbestos, 1947, 241.
57 Ibid., 109.
58 *Procès-verbal*, La ville d'Asbestos, 1947, 276; and *L'Asbestos*, August 22, 1947, 1.
59 H.R. Rice, "The Asbestos Industry in Quebec," *Canadian Mining Journal*, October 1948, 148.
60 Ibid., 159.
61 *Canadian Mining Journal*, February 1938, 65.
62 *Procès-verbal*, La ville d'Asbestos, January 24, 1949, 35.

CHAPTER 3: NEGOTIATING RISK, 1918-49

1   Schepers, "Chronology of Asbestos Cancer Discoveries," 600.
2   Robert H. Jones, *Asbestos and Asbestic*, 307.
3   This is based on extensive research of Johns-Manville corporate correspondence, wherein medical professionals stationed in Asbestos explained to officials that they did not inform workers of their diseases in order to prevent the anguish that would come from knowing they were ill. See the files at the ACRF.
4   Lankton, *Cradle to Grave*, 195.
5   Cooke, "Fibrosis of the Lungs," 487.
6   Cooke, "Pulmonary Asbestosis," 1024.
7   "Asbestos Chronology," 1929, ACRF, 4.
8   Vigod, *Quebec before Duplessis*, 134.
9   Dr. George Wright to Dr. Knight, Metropolitan Life Insurance Company, ACRF, January 19, 1925, 1.
10 Dr. Frank G. Pedley, 1929. "Doc. 7," ACRF, 3.
11 Ibid., 3.
12 Pedley, "Asbestosis," 253.
13 Egilman and Hom, "Corruption of the Medical Literature," 402.
14 Frank G. Pedley, "Report of the Physical Examination and X-Ray Examination of Asbestos Workers in Asbestos and Thetford Mines, Quebec" (Unpublished. Montreal: McGill/ Metropolitan Life, 1930), ACRF, 9.
15 Pedley, "Review of E.R.A. Merewether," 873.
16 Pedley, "Report of the Physical Examination," 9.
17 Ibid., 15–16.
18 Ibid., 16.
19 Pedley, "Asbestosis," p. 253.
20 Twenty-four out of 54 men tested at Thetford had asbestosis. Pedley, "Report of the Physical Examination," p. 10.
21 "Science Supplement," "Reviews and Retrospects," *Canadian Medical Association Journal*, 17, 1, 93; Agnew, "The Reduction of Noise in Hospitals," 417.
22 E.M. Voorhees, Johns-Manville Co., to S.A. Williams, VP Johns-Manville Co., July 28, 1931. "Asbestos Chronology," ACRF, 6.
23 Dr. McConnell, Metropolitan Life, to JM Attorneys, July 9, 1931, "Doc. 7," ACRF, 129.
24 Pedley, "Review of Studies in Experimental Pneumonokoniosis," 883.
25 Egilman, Fehnel, and Bohme, "Exposing the 'Myth' of ABC," 541.
26 Sparks, "Pulmonary Asbestosis," 1249.

27 C.H. Shoemaker, VP, C-JM Co. Asbestos, to S.A. Williams, VP, JM, December 24, 1932. "Asbestos Chronology," ACRF, 9.

28 Ibid., 9.

29 Tweedale, *Magic Mineral to Killer Dust.*

30 Merewether and Price, "A Memorandum on Asbestosis," 114.

31 Pedley, "Review of 'Pulmonary Asbestosis,'" 488.

32 Leroy Gardner to A.J. Lanza, Saranac Laboratory, April 14, 1933. "Doc. 7," ACRF, 79.

33 Vandiver Brown, JM VP, to Lewis H. Brown, JM President, May 10, 1933. "Asbestos Chronology," ACRF, 11.

34 A.J. Lanza, Proceedings of the Home Office Underwriters Association, November 1933. "Doc. 7," ACRF, 10.

35 See, for example, A.J. Lanza, "Asbestosis," *Journal of the American Medical Association* 106, 5 (1936): 368–69.

36 Minutes of a meeting between Johns-Manville Co., Raybestos-Manhattan Co., and Metropolitan Life, December 29, 1933. "Asbestos Chronology," ACRF, 13.

37 Vandiver Brown, VP JM, internal memo, January 15, 1935. "Doc. 7," ACRF, 6.

38 Sumner Simpson, President, Raybestos-Manhattan, to Vandiver Brown, VP JM, October 1, 1935. "Asbestos Chronology," ACRF, 18.

39 Vandiver Brown, VP JM, to Dr. L. Gardner, Saranac Laboratory, November 20, 1936. "Doc. 7," ACRF, 89.

40 Sumner Simpson, President, Raybestos-Manhattan, to Schluter, November 10, 1936. "Doc. 7," ACRF, 82.

41 Kesteman, Southam, and Saint-Pierre, *Histoire des Cantons de l'est*, 563.

42 R.H. Stevenson, C-JM Asbestos, "Talk by Dr. Stevenson to Quebec Asbestos Producers," May 23, 1938, Turner & Newall Archives, 1.

43 Ibid., 1.

44 Ibid., 1.

45 C.S. Bell, Esq., to Sir Samuel Turner, President, Turner & Newall, July 4, 1938, Turner & Newall Archives 1.

46 JM Board of Directors Meeting Minutes, April 18, 1938. "Asbestos Chronology," ACRF, 21.

47 JM Internal Memo, September 1938. "Asbestos Chronology," ACRF, 22.

48 JM Internal Memo, September 1938. "Asbestos Chronology," ACRF, 22.

49 "Asbestos Chronology," 1939, ACRF, 23.

50 "Hospital Equipment and Accident Prevention at Asbestos, Que. Take Hazards out of Industry," "Asbestos Chronology," 1939, ACRF, 22.

51 Ibid., 22.

52 R.H. Stevenson, "Asbestosis," 1940, Turner & Newall Archives, 1.

53 Ibid., 2.

54 Ibid., 4.

55 Ibid., 4.

56 Ibid., 5.

57 Ibid., 5.

58 Ibid., 1.

59 Ibid., 8.

60 F. Bussy, Turner & Newall Co., to W.W.F. Shepherd, Turner & Newall Co., May 25, 1940, Turner & Newall Archives, 1.

61 Greenberg, "A Report," 235–36.

62 A.R. Fisher, JM, to J.P. Woodard, Attorney, JM, June 29, 1945. "Asbestos Chronology," ACRF, 37.

63 MacDermot, *History of the CMA*, vol. 2, 138–39.

64 R. Desmeules et al., "Amiantose et Cancers Pulmonaires," 99–105.

65 Ibid., 97.

66 Ibid., 108.

67 Ibid., 108.

68 Dr. Leroy Gardner, Saranac Laboratory, to Hektoen, JM, March 15, 1943. "Doc. 7," ACRF, 31; Dr. Leroy Gardner, "Draft Report," "Doc. 7," ACRF, 29.

69 Dr. Leroy Gardner, Saranac Laboratory, to Vandiver Brown, VP JM, February 24, 1943. "Asbestos Chronology," ACRF, 30.

70 Rousseau, "Amiantose Pulmonaire," 239.

71 Ibid., 238.

72 This is based on a thorough study of every issue of *Laval Medical* printed, which shows a marked increase in the number of publications on asbestos-related disease during the mid-1940s.

73 H.K. Sherry, President C-JM, memo, May 24, 1944. "Asbestos Chronology," ACRF, 33.

74 Leroy Gardner, Saranac Laboratory, to Vandiver Brown, VP JM, July 15, 1944. "Asbestos Chronology," ACRF, 33.

75 G.K. Foster, C-JM, memo to A.R. Fisher, C-JM, August 9, 1944. "Asbestos Chronology," ACRF, 34.

76 Ibid., 34.

77 McCulloch and Tweedale, *Defending the Indefensible*, 28.

78 Joan Ross, "Survey of Female Employees in Canadian Textile Department," 1944. "Asbestos Chronology," ACRF, 34.

79 Ibid., 34.

80 October 27, 1944. "Asbestos Chronology," ACRF, 35.

81 Rousseau, "Quelque considérations," 66.

82 Vandiver Brown memo, 1947, "Asbestos Chronology," ACRF 39; Vandiver Brown, VP JM, to J.P. Woodard, JM, March 21, 1947. "Asbestos Chronology," ACRF, 40.

83 See, for example, D.S. Egbert and A.J. Geiger, "Pulmonary Asbestosis and Carcinoma," *American Review of Tuberculosis* 34 (1936), 143–50; M. Nordmann, "The Occupational Cancer of Asbestos Workers," *Z Krebsforsch* 47 (1938), 288–302; and E.R.A. Merewether, *Annual Report of the Chief Inspector of Factories for the Year 1947*, Great Britain. For more information on the early links between asbestos and cancer, see, Barry I. Castleman, "Letter to the Editor," *British Journal of Industrial Medicine* 48 (1991): 427–30.

84 A.R. Fisher, JM, to J.P. Woodard, JM, July 22, 1947. "Asbestos Chronology," ACRF, 41.

85 "Tuberculose et Amiantose," *Laval médical* 12, 8 (1947): 1090.

86 Kenneth Smith, C-JM Asbestos, to H.F. Janson, Department Supervisor, Mill, C-JM Asbestos, January 21, 1947. "Asbestos Chronology," ACRF, 39.

87 Kenneth Smith, C-JM Asbestos, to Ivan Sabourin, JM, March 13, 1947. "Asbestos Chronology," ACRF, 40.

88 Kenneth Smith, C-JM Asbestos, to Paul Cartier, Thetford, September 11, 1947. "Asbestos Chronology," ACRF, 41.

89 In March 1948, Smith supplied two visiting doctors with files of employees he had already deemed healthy. Writing of his deception to Cartier, Smith stated, "we never have let anyone know that this company (JM) had anything to do with the scheme; we are merely

co-operating with … the Board to the best of our ability … Even the head of the union here thinks that." See Kenneth Smith, C-JM Asbestos, to Paul Cartier, Thetford, July 6, 1948. "Asbestos Chronology," ACRF, 43.

90 Vandiver Brown, VP JM, to Ernest Muehleck (Keasby & Mattison) and Rohrbach, Raybestos-Manhattan, October 22, 1948. "Asbestos Chronology," ACRF, 47.

91 Ibid.

92 Kenneth Smith, C-JM Asbestos, to J.E. Morrison, C-JM Asbestos, December 1, 1948. "Asbestos Chronology," ACRF, 47.

93 H. Jackson, C-JM Asbestos, to J.E. Morrison, C-JM Asbestos, December 6, 1948. "Asbestos Chronology," ACRF, 47–48.

94 Kenneth Smith, C-JM Asbestos, to G.K. Foster, President, C-JM Asbestos, December 6, 1948. "Asbestos Chronology," ACRF, 47.

95 LeDoux, *L'Amiantose à East Broughton*, 3.

96 Ibid., 5.

97 Ibid., 5.

98 Ibid., 5.

99 Ibid., 6.

100 "L'AMIANTOSE EST INCURABLE, MAIS ON PEUT LA PREVENIR," English translation by author, Ibid., 8.

101 *L'Asbestos*, January 1949, and LeDoux, 58–60.

Chapter 4: Essential Characteristics, 1918-49

1 Frederic Tomesco, "Asbestos, Quebec, Seeks a Healthier Name Not Linked to Cancer," *Bloomberg,* July 14, 2006, http://www.bloomberg.com/apps/news?pid=newsarchive&refer=canada&sid=acD5eSZMS.rc.

2 Ibid.

3 *Canadian Mining Journal*, February 5, 1919, 66.

4 "Une Grève se Déclare dans les Mines de la Manville Asbestos Co.," *La Tribune*, May 29, 1918, 1.

5 *Procès-verbal*, La ville d'Asbestos, June 4, 1919, 189–97.

6 Asbestos paid JM a percentage of the cost it took to run the electricity and a percentage of the profits gained from it until 1929. *Procès-verbal*, La ville d'Asbestos, July 23, 1919, 200.

7 Ewen, "The International Unions," 127; Heron, *The Canadian Labour Movement*, 53.

8 "Formation d'une Union Ouvrière à Asbestos," *La Tribune*, October 15, 1919, 1.

9 Denis, "The Mining Industry," 4.

10 Kesteman, Southam, and Saint-Pierre, *Histoire des Cantons de l'Est*, 276, 490.

11 Vallières, *Des Mines et des Hommes*, 215.

12 *Canadian Mining Journal*, August 5, 1921, 619.

13 *Canadian Mining Journal*, January 28, 1921, 63.

14 Rouillard, *Le Syndicalisme Québécois*, 40.

15 Rouillard, *Les Syndicats Nationaux*, 223, 225, 227.

16 Industrial relations in Quebec's asbestos industry had changed since 1918, and when Thetford workers went on strike in 1921, new employees replaced the miners who attempted to hold out for a raise.

17 Letter from the Deputy Minister of Labour to "Sir," "Strike 22, April 1923," Department of Labour, Strikes and Lockouts, LAC, RG 27, Vol. 330, Reel T-2713, 5; *Ottawa Journal*, April 27, 1923, "Strike 22, April 1923," Department of Labour, Strikes and Lockouts, LAC, RG 27, Vol. 330, Reel T-2713.

18 Kesteman, Southam, and Saint-Pierre, *Histoire des Cantons de l'Est*, 541.

19 *Procès-verbal*, La ville d'Asbestos, February 5, 1925, 6.

20 *Procès-verbal*, La ville d'Asbestos, August 11, 1927, 151; December 31, 1928, 229.

21 *Procès-verbal*, La ville d'Asbestos, June 2, 1927, 6–7.

22 Gray, "Asbestos Industry Readjusted," 402.

23 McCulloch and Tweedale, *Defending the Indefensible*, 25.

24 *Procès-verbal*, La ville d'Asbestos, January 25, 1932, 435.

25 *Procès-verbal*, La ville d'Asbestos, December 6, 1933, 146.

26 *Procès-verbal*, La ville d'Asbestos, February 21, 1934, 168.

27 *Procès-verbal*, La ville d'Asbestos, March 7, 1934, 171.

28 *Procès-verbal*, La ville d'Asbestos, July 16, 1934, 211.

29 Jones, *Duplessis and the Union Nationale Administration*, 5.

30 Vallières, *Des Mines et des Hommes*, 215.

31 Strike Report, March 27, 1937. Department of Labour, Strikes and Lockouts, LAC, RG 27, vol. 330, Reel T-2713; H.K. Sherry, Strike Report, February 2, 1937, Department of Labour, Strikes and Lockouts, LAC, RG 27, vol. 330, Reel T-2713, 8.

32 *Toronto Clarion*, January 27, 1937. Department of Labour, Strikes and Lockouts, LAC, RG 27, vol. 330, Reel T-2713, 29.

33 *The Gazette* (Montreal), January 26, 1937. Department of Labour, Strikes and Lockouts, LAC, RG 27, vol. 330, Reel T-2713, 31.

34 *The Gazette* (Montreal), January 27, 1937. Department of Labour, Strikes and Lockouts, LAC, RG 27, vol. 330, Reel T-2713, 28.

35 *Toronto Telegram*, January 29, 1937. Department of Labour, Strikes and Lockouts, LAC, RG 27, vol. 330, Reel T-2713, 23.

36 *Winnipeg Manitoba Commonwealth*, February 19, 1937. Department of Labour, Strikes and Lockouts, LAC, RG 27, vol. 330, Reel T-2713, 4.

37 Lewis H. Brown, JM President, to Olive Cry, President of the National Catholic Syndicat, Asbestos, PQ, January 29, 1937; *Toronto Telegram*, January 29, 1937. Department of Labour, Strikes and Lockouts, LAC, RG 27, vol. 330, Reel T-2713, 9.

38 *Quebec Chronicle Telegram*, March 24, 1937. Department of Labour, Strikes and Lockouts, LAC, RG 27, vol. 330, Reel T-2713, 2.

39 For more information on the Padlock Law and the policies of Duplessis, please see *Le Rouge et le Bleu: Une anthologie de la pensée politique au Québec de la Conquête à la Révolution tranquille*, ed. Yvan Lamonde and Claude Corbo (Montreal: Les Presses de l'université de Montréal, 1999), 427.

40 A.O. Dufresne, C-JM Director, to "Gentlemen," February 14, 1938. BANQ, P182 3A 017 03–01–003B-01; 2000–10–013\3.

41 *Johns-Manville Photo*, December 1938, 2.

42 *Johns-Manville Photo*, June 1939, 2.

43 *Johns-Manville Photo*, October 1940, 2.

44 "For Release: Director of Public Information," April 26, 1940, 2; August 16, 1940, 3; September 27, 1940, 4. BANQ, "Industries de Guerre," E8 7A 021 03–05–001B-01; 1960–01–040\183 e24.

45 Oliver Bowles and K.G. Warner, "Asbestos," *Minerals Yearbook 1939*, ed. Herbert Hughes (Washington: US GPO, 1939), 1310.

46 *Le Citoyen*, December 28, 1974, 97.

47 Rouillard, *Le Syndicalisme Québécois*, 130.

48 *Johns-Manville Photo*, September 1944 2; *L'Asbestos*, April 7, 1943, 1.

49 *L'Asbestos*, February 17, 1943, 3.

50 Linteau et al, *Quebec Since 1930*, 222.

51 Gérard Pelletier, "Témoignages," in Gagnon and Sarra-Bournet, eds., *Duplessis*, 23.

52 R.L. Bruneau, Manager, Unemployment Insurance Commission, to Mr. MacLean, Director of Industrial Relations, Department of Labour, Ottawa, March 22, 1945; RG 27, Vol. 440, Reel T-4072, LAC, 4; Strike Report, March 27, 1945. "Strike 53, March 1945," Department of Labour, Strikes and Lockouts, LAC, RG 27, vol. 440, Reel T-4072, 1.

53 C.M. McGaw, C-JM, Strike Report, November 28, 1945. "Strike 197, November 1945," Department of Labour, Strikes and Lockouts, LAC, RG 27, vol. 443, Reel T-4076, 1–2.

54 Strike Report, January 26, 1946. "Strike 3, January 1946," Department of Labour, Strikes and Lockouts, LAC, RG 27, vol. 444, Reel T-4076, 3.

55 R.L. Bruneau, Manager, "Summary," January 16, 1946. RG 27, Vol. 444, Reel T-4076, LAC, 9.

56 R.L. Bruneau, "Report on Industrial Dispute," May 3, 1946. "Strike 71, May 1946," Department of Labour, Strikes and Lockouts, LAC, RG 27, vol. 445, Reel T-4077, 5.

57 "Johns Manville Annual Report, 1948," seen in McCulloch and Tweedale, *Defending the Indefensible*, 30.

58 Report on Strike, January 20, 1948. "Strike 1, January 1948," Department of Labour, Strikes and Lockouts, LAC, RG 27, vol. 461, Reel T-4092, , 1–2.

59 *L'Asbestos*, April 16, 1948, 1.

60 Gérard Tremblay, Quebec Deputy Minister of Labour, to Paul E. Bernier, Secretary, Commission de Relations ouvrières, April 21, 1948; and Gérard Tremblay, Quebec Deputy Minister of Labour, to Cyprien Miron, Director, Service de conciliation et d'arbitrage, April 21, 1948, BANQ, P659 7C 018 05–02–008B-01; 1982–11–008\1.

61 *L'Asbestos*, April 23, 1948, 1.

62 *L'Asbestos*, April 30, 1948, 1 and 5.

63 Cyprien Miron, Director, Service de conciliation et d'arbitrage, to Gérard Tremblay, Quebec Deputy Minister of Labour, May 10, 1948, BANQ, P659 7C 018 05–02–008B-01; 1982–11–008\1.

64 *L'Asbestos*, May 14, 1948. Department capitalized in official documents.

65 Armand Larivée, SNA President, to Albert Goudreau, MLA, June 19, 1948, BANQ, P659 7C 018 05–02–008B-01; 1982–11–008\1.

66 Barrette, *Memoirs*, 100.

67 *L'Asbestos*, January 14, 1949, 1.

68 "Renseignements qui doivent accompagner une requite pour intervention conciliatrice en vertu des dispositions de l'article 13 de la loi des relations ouvrieres de la province," Intervention Paper, January 31, 1949, BANQ, P659 7C 018 05–02–008B-01; 1982–11–008\1.

69 G.K. Foster, C-JM, to Antonio Barrette, Quebec Minister of Labour, January 31, 1949, BANQ, P659 7C 018 05–02–008B-01; 1982–11–008\1.

CHAPTER 5: BODIES COLLIDE

1 For in-depth studies on this, see Behiels, *Prelude to Quebec's Quiet Revolution*; and McRoberts, *Quebec*.
2 See Letourneau, "La grève de l'amiante," in which he describes the difficulty in getting people in Asbestos to discuss the strike.
3 Antonio Barrette, Quebec Minister of Labour, to Jean Marchand, Secretary of the CTCC and Rodolphe Hamel, President of the SNA, n.d., BANQ, P182 3 A017 03–01–003B-01; 2000–10–013\3.
4 *Johns-Manville News Pictorial*, January 1949, 6–7.
5 *La Tribune*, February 15, 1949 5.
6 "Si tu as ta brosse à dents, ca suffit. Tu n'as même pas besoin d'un pyjama; cette grève ne durera pas 48 heures," English translation by author, Gérard Pelletier, *Le Citoyen*, December 28, 1974, 114.
7 This is possibly because his criticism of Duplessis and his later career as a federal Liberal cabinet minister led scholars to interpret his reports as simply yet another intellectual attack on the government's conservative hold on the province. See, for example, Black, *Duplessis*, 521.
8 *La Tribune*, February 15, 1949, 5; Gérard Pelletier, "The Strike and the Press," in Trudeau, *The Asbestos Strike*, 243.
9 *La Tribune*, February 15, 1949, 5; *L'Asbestos*, February 18, 1949, 1.
10 *L'Asbestos*, February 18, 1949, 1; *La Tribune*, February 19, 1949, 1.
11 C-JM to Antonio Barrette and Maurice Duplessis, February 18, 1949, BANQ, P182 3 A017 03–01–003B-01; 2000–10–013\3.
12 *Le Devoir*, February 23, 1949, 1.
13 "S'ils viennent, c'est alors que cela va aller mal ... Les grévistes sont paisibles et ils n'ont fait aucun dommage à la propriété," *La Tribune*, February 21, 1949, 1; "considérée à Asbestos comme un geste de méfiance que rien ne justifie," English translations by author, *Le Devoir*, February 21, 1949, 2.
14 *La Tribune*, February 23, 1949, 3.
15 *Procès-verbal*, La ville d'Asbestos, February 21, 1949, 38.
16 See, for example, "Police Drunk, Indecent, Caused First Disorders, Asbestos Council Says," *Globe and Mail*, February 22, 1949, 11; *Toronto Star*, February 21, 1949, 11, 14.
17 *Globe and Mail*, February 23, 1949, 10.
18 *Le Devoir*, February 23, 1949, 3.
19 "très heureux de vivre avec de tels sauvages," English translation by author, Ibid., 3.
20 *L'Asbestos*, February 25, 1949, 1; *Le Devoir*, February 25, 1949, 3; *La Tribune*, March 1, 1949, 5.
21 *L'Asbestos*, March 4, 1949, 1.
22 *Le Devoir*, March 3, 1949, 3.
23 *La Tribune*, March 4, 1949, 3.
24 *Le Devoir*, March 7, 1949, 3.
25 "plus graves, moins légers, après ces trois semaines de grève," English translation by author, Ibid., 3.
26 *Le Devoir*, March 8, 1949, 1.
27 *L'Asbestos*, March 11, 1949, 1.

28 *Le Devoir*, March 14, 1949, 3.
29 *L'Asbestos*, March 7, 1949, 6. Before the strike, Jeffrey Mine workers earned 85 cents an hour and typically worked eight-hour shifts each day.
30 Ibid., 1.
31 *Le Devoir*, March 12, 1949, 3.
32 *La Tribune*, March 15, 1949, 3.
33 *L'Asbestos*, March 18, 1949, 1.
34 *La Tribune*, March 17, 1949, 1.
35 Ibid., 1.
36 *L'Asbestos*, March 18, 1949, 5–6.
37 *Le Devoir*, March 19, 1949, 3.
38 Kenneth Smith to G.K. Foster, C-JM President, March 19, 1949. "Asbestos Chronology," ACRF, 50.
39 *Le Devoir*, March 19, 1949, 3.
40 "casser le gueule au curé," English translation by author, *La Tribune*, March 21, 1949, 3.
41 It is unclear whether Roger Beauchemin was related to Paul Beauchemin, the nonunionized worker mentioned above, who had been beaten. In a community as small as Asbestos, it is likely that they were related in some way. *Le Devoir*, March 22, 1949, 1.
42 "j'aurais pas cru qu'on trouvait des hommes pour des ouvrages sales comme celui-là," English translation by author, *Le Devoir*, March 23, 1949, 3.
43 "si j'étais mineur, je serais moi-même en grève et dans les circonstances, j'aurais la conscience parfaitement tranquille," English translation by author, Ibid., 2.
44 *L'Asbestos*, April 1, 1949, 4.
45 *La Tribune*, March 25, 1949, 3.
46 *La Tribune*, March 26, 1949, 1.
47 *La Tribune*, March 31, 1949, April 2 and 3, 1949, 3.
48 "Pas de contrat, pas de travail," "Notre grève est juste et morale," "Vive la police provinciale," and "Qui a fait sauter les rails?" English translation by author, *Le Devoir*, April 4, 1949, 3.
49 "L'amiante-jeu," at the Société d'Histoire d'Asbestos. The Société does not have numbers cataloguing its collection.
50 *La Tribune*, April 8, 1949, 1.
51 *Globe and Mail*, April 12, 1949, 10.
52 *La Tribune*, April 11, 1949, 1.
53 "à faire un peu de poussière," English translation by author, *Le Devoir*, April 14, 1949, 3.
54 J.P. Woodard, JM lawyer, to G.K. Foster, President, C-JM, 15 April 1949. "Asbestos Chronology," ACRF, 47.
55 *L'Asbestos*, April 15, 1949, 2.
56 *La Tribune*, April 18, 1949, 1.
57 "le terreur qui régne," English translation by author, *Le Devoir*, April 18, 1949, 3.
58 *La Tribune*, April 19, 1949, 1.
59 Kenneth Smith, statement to the press, April 20, 1949. "Asbestos Chronology," ACRF, 47.
60 G.K. Foster, C-JM President, to Antonio Barrette, Quebec Minister of Labour, April 21, 1949, BANQ, P182 3 A017 03–01–003B-01; 2000–10–013\3.
61 "Une gréviste d'Asbestos" to Prime Minister Louis St-Laurent, April 22, 1949. LAC, MG 26-L, vol. 56, file I-25–3-A, 1949, pp. 1–2.
62 *Le Devoir*, April 22, 1949, 3. Because of the CTCC's religious affiliation, local priests were part of each chapter's administration.

63   *La Tribune*, April 22, 1949, 1.

64   *La Tribune*, April 21, 1949, 3.

65   *Globe and Mail*, April 23, 1949, 7.

66   *La Tribune*, April 25, 1949, 1.

67   *Procès-verbal*, La ville d'Asbestos, April 26, 1949, 50.

68   *Le Devoir*, April 29, 1949, 3.

69   *Procès-verbal*, La ville d'Asbestos, April 29, 1949, 51.

70   *Johns-Manville News Pictorial*, May 1949, 3.

71   *La Patrie*, May 2, 1949, 1.

72   *Le Devoir*, May 2, 1949, 3.

73   *Procès-verbal*, La ville d'Asbestos, May 2, 1949, 53.

74   *Le Devoir*, May 4, 1949, 3.

75   *Le Devoir*, May 5, 1949, 3.

76   *Globe and Mail*, May 6, 1949, 1.

77   Ibid., 1.

78   *Globe and Mail*, May 7, 1949, 2.

79   Gérard Pelletier, "The Strike and the Press," in Trudeau, *The Asbestos Strike*, 264.

80   Ibid., 264.

81   Ibid., 264.

82   "maîtres de la situation," English translation by author, *Le Devoir*, May 6, 1949, 3; *La Tribune*, May 6, 1949, 1.

83   *La Tribune*, May 5, 1949, 1.

84   *Le Devoir*, May 6, 1949, 3.

85   *Globe and Mail*, May 7, 1949, 2.

86   *L'Asbestos*, May 6, 1949, 1.

87   "Testimony of Joseph Beaudoin," *Declarations sur la Brutalité*, 12; "Testimony of Bruno Champagne," *Declarations sur la Brutalité*, 17.

88   "Testimony of Gérard Chamberland, *Declarations sur la Brutalité*, 7.

89   "Testimony of Emile Grimard," *Declarations sur la Brutalité*, 11; "Testimony of Alfred Blanchette," *Declarations sur la Brutalité*, 1.

90   "Testimony of Jean-Paul Houle," *Declarations sur la Brutalité*, 15.

91   *La Tribune*, May 7, 1949, 3.

92   *Globe and Mail*, May 7, 1949, 1–2; *Le Devoir*, May 7, 1949, 2.

93   "malaise et l'amertume," English translation by author, *La Tribune*, May 7, 1949, 1.

94   *La Presse*, May 7, 1949, 1.

95   *Globe and Mail*, May 9, 1949, 1.

96   Ibid., 1. Jean Drapeau would later become mayor of Montreal.

97   *Le Devoir*, May 10, 1949, 10.

98   Brown, "La Grève d'Asbestos," 15.

99   Ibid., 15.

100   *Le Devoir*, May 11, 1949, 3.

101   "Désolation règne à Asbestos," English translation by author, *L'Asbestos*, May 13, 1949, 1.

102   *La Tribune*, May 16, 1949, 1; May 31, 1949, 1.

103   Paul Parrott, demographer, to W.H. Soutar, C-JM Assistant Mine Manager, May 24, 1949, "Asbestos Chronology," ACRF, 51.

104   June 15, 1949, "Asbestos Chronology," ACRF, 47.

105   *La Tribune*, May 27, 1949, 3.

106 "Asbestos Production Limited as Strike Continues," *Johns-Manville News Pictorial*, June 1949, 2.
107 *Le Devoir*, June 20, 1949, 1.
108 *Globe and Mail*, June 23, 1949, 1.
109 *Procès-verbal*, La ville d'Asbestos, June 22, 1949, 61.
110 *Le Devoir*, June 25, 1949, 1.
111 *Le Devoir*, July 1, 1949, 1.
112 *Le Devoir*, July 1, 1949, 1.
113 *L'Asbestos*, June 30, 1949, 1.

CHAPTER 6 : "UNE VILLE QUI SE DEPLACE"

1 *Entre Nous*, February 1951, 8.
2 Josephson and Barsigian, "Asbestos," 139; *Canadian Mining Journal*, August 1949, 54.
3 *Procès-verbal*, La ville d'Asbestos, August 3, 1949, 67–68.
4 *Procès-verbal*, La ville d'Asbestos, September 9, 1949, 73; June 7, 1950, 138.
5 *Procès-verbal*, La ville d'Asbestos, August 9, 1950, 154; October 4, 1950, 164.
6 *United States Geological Survey 1950* (Washington: US GPO, 1951): 6.
7 "Asbestos: Where We Live and Work," *Johns-Manville News Pictorial* (October 1950), 8.
8 Vallières, *Des Mines et des Hommes*, 348.
9 *Entre Nous*, February 1951, 9.
10 This information was taken from a USGS report on a 1952 visit to Asbestos to survey operations. *United States Geological Survey 1952* (Washington: US GPO, 1953): III–2.
11 *Canadian Mining Journal*, February 1952, 106.
12 *Johns-Manville News Pictorial*, July 1953, 3.
13 *Procès-verbal*, La ville d'Asbestos, September 2, 1953, 73.
14 Walkom, "New Shaft," 57.
15 Ibid., 58.
16 *Canadian Mining Journal*, February 1955, 89–90.
17 *Procès-verbal*, La ville d'Asbestos, July 21, 1955, 236.
18 *Le Citoyen*, October 7, 1955, 1
19 *Le Citoyen*, July 26, 1956, 2.
20 *Canadian Mining Journal*, February 1957, 107; *Le Citoyen*, December 20, 1957, 1. The company made more than $100,000,000 in 1957.
21 *Procès-verbal*, La ville d'Asbestos, May 20, 1958, 174.
22 *Le Citoyen*, July 25, 1958, 1; April 17, 1959, 1.
23 *Procès-verbal*, La ville d'Asbestos, May 27, 1958, 176.
24 *Le Citoyen*, May 15, 1959, 1.
25 *Procès-verbal*, La ville d'Asbestos, September 19, 1959, pp. 48–49.
26 *Canadian Mining Journal*, February 1960, 160.
27 "Asbestos doit produire plus d'amiante," (author's English translation), *Le Citoyen*, March 18, 1960, 1.
28 *Canadian Mining Journal*, February 1962, 117.
29 *Le Citoyen*, January 30, 1964, 1.
30 The local paper in Asbestos had been renamed *Le Citoyen* in 1950 although it remained under the same editorial board. Ibid., 1.
31 *Le Citoyen*, February 13, 1964, 1.

32 "bouge au Québec," English translation by author, *Le Citoyen*, October 14, 1964, 4.

33 Hansard. Journal des débats de l'Assemblée législative, 27ᵉ législature, 3ᵉ session (14 janvier 1964 au 31 juillet 1964), Le vendredi 19 juin 1964 – Vol. 1 N° 96.

34 *Procès-verbal*, La ville d'Asbestos, November 4, 1964, 7.

35 "une ville qui se deplace," English translation by author, *Le Citoyen*, December 19, 1964, 4.

36 Antonio Hamel to Bérubé, Government of Quebec, October 10, 1979, BANQ, E78 S999, 7 A 009 03–06–004B-01; 1993–06–004\12.

37 Ross, "Encroachment of the Jeffrey Mine," 534.

38 Ibid.

39 *Canadian Mining Journal*, May 1967, 45.

40 "Amiante: Notre Patrimoine," translation by author, *Le Citoyen*, December 28, 1974, 186.

41 "nous en avons soupé de la poussière et du bruit," English translation by author, *Le Citoyen*, April 23, 1968, 1.

42 *Procès-verbal*, La ville d'Asbestos, April 17, 1968, 62.

43 *Procès-verbal*, La ville d'Asbestos, October 2, 1968 117 and March 5, 1969, 180.

44 *Procès-verbal*, La ville d'Asbestos, September 29, 1969, 250.

45 *Le Citoyen*, December 22, 1970, 1.

46 *Le Citoyen*, January 26, 1971, 1; *Procès-verbal*, La ville d'Asbestos, February 10, 1971.

47 *Procès-verbal*, La ville d'Asbestos, September 27, 1971.

48 *Canadian Mining Journal*, February 1972, 139.

49 "mauvaise mine," English translation by author, *Le Citoyen*, January 28, 1975, 4.

50 "Mais, pour aller où?," English translation by author, *Le Citoyen*, April 15, 1975, 3.

51 *Le Citoyen*, February 4, 1975, 3.

52 June 5, 1975, BANQ, E78 S999, 7D 024 02–01–001A-01; 1985–02–006\2.

53 Yves Hamel, Asbestos, to Yves Bérubé, Quebec MNR, October 10, 1979, BANQ, E78 S999, 7D 024 02–01–001A-01; 1985–02–006\2.

54 *Canadian Mining Journal*, February 1977, 125.

55 *Procès-verbal*, La ville d'Asbestos, May 18, 1977.

56 Fish, "Canadian Johns-Manville," 8.

57 Ibid., 11.

58 *Procès-verbal*, La ville d'Asbestos, January 18, 1978.

59 Gérard Piché, C-JM Administrative Services to Marie Fortin-Drouin, September 1979, BANQ, E78 S999, 7D 024 02–01–001A-01; 1985–02–006\2.

60 Desrochers to Government of Quebec, September 1979, BANQ, E78 S999, 7D 024 02–01–001A-01; 1985–02–006\2.

61 *Procès-verbal*, La ville d'Asbestos, September, 17, 1980, 109.

62 *Canadian Mining Journal*, February 1981, 129.

63 "working crater," translation by author, *Procès-verbal*, La ville d'Asbestos, January 21, 1981, 171.

64 *Procès-verbal*, La ville d'Asbestos, May 5, 1981, 222.

65 *Procès-verbal*, La ville d'Asbestos, May 19, 1981, 235; *Canadian Mining Journal*, February 1982, 122.

66 *Procès-verbal*, La ville d'Asbestos, June 1, 1982, 156.

67 *Le Citoyen*, August 10, 1982, 2.

68 *Canadian Mining Journal*, February 1983, 100.

69 This name was taken from a long-standing nickname for the mineral, which was "white gold," because chrysotile asbestos was white in colour and worth just as much as, if not more than, gold. *Procès-verbal*, La ville d'Asbestos, May 17, 1968, 73.

70 "il apparaissait très clair que l'âge d'or de l'amiante était terminé et qu'une nouvelle bataille s'annonçait, plus difficile encore, pour la survie de la communauté et de son industrie centenaire." Translation by author. Lampron, Cantin, and Grimard, *Asbestos*, 335.

71 "Usant d'une imagination toujours plus aiguë pour dynamiser et revivifier une communauté qui en a bien besoin, la Ville se démènera avec une énergie insoupçonnée afin de conserver ce qui lui reste: son âme." Translation by author. Ibid.

72 *Procès-verbal*, La ville d'Asbestos, December 6, 1983, 135.

73 Vagt, "Asbestos," 143.

74 *Procès-verbal*, La ville d'Asbestos, December 19, 1983, 143.

75 BANQ, E78 S999 2A 026 02–05–004A-01; 1993–05–005\4 6.

Chapter 7: Useful Tools, 1949-83

1 "on peut vivre en vainqueur," English translation by author, *Globe and Mail*, March 31, 1997, A4; Dolbec, "Les marathoniens," A2.

2 Institut National de Santé Publique du Québec, "The Epidemiology of Asbestos-Related Diseases in Quebec" (Quebec: Insitut National de Santé Publique du Québec, 2004): 53.

3 See, for example, Buckley, *Danger, Death and Disaster*, 144.

4 "Asbestos Chronology," ACRF, 1949, 46.

5 Author unknown. Gatke Corporation to Vandiver Brown, JM VP, "Doc 7," ACRF, June 1949, 34.

6 Kenneth Smith, "Unpublished Report: Survey of Men in Dusty Areas," "Doc 7," ACRF 16.

7 Ibid., 3.

8 Kenneth Smith, "Industrial Hygiene – Survey of Men in Dusty Areas," 1949, "Asbestos Chronology," ACRF, 46.

9 J.P. Woodard, JM, to L.C. Bart, JM, August 8, 1949, "Asbestos Chronology," ACRF, 49.

10 C.M. McGaw, C-JM, to C.W. Hite, JM, August 1949, "Asbestos Chronology," ACRF, 49.

11 J.P. Woodard, JM Attorney, to M.C. McGaw, C-JM, August 18, 1949, "Asbestos Chronology," ACRF, 52.

12 Testimony of John Vorwald in Arbitration of the Asbestos Strike, 1949, as seen in Tataryn, *Dying for a Living*, 28.

13 John Vorwald, Saranac Laboratories, to Kenneth Smith, C-JM, October 15, 1949, "Asbestos Chronology," ACRF, 50.

14 *Le Devoir*, December 15, 1949, 1.

15 This included new studies by E.R.A. Merewether in Great Britain. Kenneth Smith to K.V. Lindell, C-JM President, January 28, 1950. "Asbestos Chronology," ACRF, 53.

16 Ibid., 53.

17 J.P. Woodard, JM Attorney, to H.H. Peterson, February 3, 1950, "Asbestos Chronology," ACRF, 51; Paul Cartier to John Vorwald, January 30, 1950, "Asbestos Chronology," ACRF, 50.

18 Kenneth Smith to J.P. Woodard, JM Attorney, February 7, 1950, "Asbestos Chronology," ACRF, 51; J.P. Woodard, JM Attorney to Kenneth Smith, March 3, 1950, "Asbestos Chronology," ACRF, 62.

19 John Vorwald to Kenneth Smith, April 18, 1950, "Asbestos Chronology," ACRF, 52.

20 For more information on the tobacco industry's attempts to control information on the dangers of cigarettes, see Peter Boyle, Nigel Gray, Jack Henningfield, John Seffrin, and

Witold A. Zatonski, eds., *Tobacco: Science, Policy, and Public Health*, 2nd ed. (Oxford: Oxford University Press, 2010).

21 Maurice Duplessis, Premier of Quebec, "Letter of Address to the Documentation catholique de Paris," May 1950, as seen in Delisle and Malouf, *Le Quatuor d'Asbestos*, 11.

22 "Asbestos for Heart Trouble," 3.

23 John Vorwald to J.P. Woodard, JM Attorney, July 25, 1950, "Asbestos Chronology," ACRF, 54.

24 Vandiver Brown, JM VP, to J.P. Woodard, JM Attorney, November 15, 1950, "Asbestos Chronology," ACRF, 56.

25 Kenneth Smith to H.M. Jackson, JM, December 19, 1950, "Asbestos Chronology," ACRF, 57.

26 C.W. McGaw, C-JM, to H.M. Jackson, 1951, "Asbestos Chronology," ACRF, 61.

27 J.P. Woodard, C.W. McGaw, H.M. Jackson, and N.S. Deeley Correspondence, January 17, 1951, "Asbestos Chronology," ACRF, 62; Kenneth Smith to C.W. McGaw, June 11, 1951, "Asbestos Chronology," ACRF, 60.

28 "JM Memorandum on History of JM Medical Program at Asbestos," October 19, 1951, "Asbestos Chronology," ACRF, 61–62.

29 1952, "Asbestos Chronology," ACRF, 62.

30 First Interim Report, May 7, 1952, "Asbestos Chronology," ACRF, 64.

31 A.J. Lanza, 1952, "Doc 7," ACRF, 9.

32 John Knox, "Visit to Thetford Mines and Asbestos," September 30, 1952, QAMA, 2.

33 Ibid., 2.

34 "Health of Employees at C-JM," 1953, "Asbestos Chronology," ACRF, 68.

35 I.H. Sloane to H.M. Jackson, April 25, 1954, "Asbestos Chronology," ACRF, 74.

36 For example, see Hueper, "Silicosis, Asbestosis, and Cancer of the Lung."

37 Richard Doll, "Mortality from Lung Cancer in Asbestos Workers," *British Journal of Industrial Medicine* 12 (1953): 86.

38 Barry I. Castleman, Asbestos: Medical and Legal Aspects, 5th edition (New York: Aspen Publishers, 2005), 83.

39 Doll, "Mortality from Lung Cancer," 86.

40 Smith, "Pulmonary Disability in Asbestos Workers," 200.

41 Ibid., 199–200.

42 J.D.M., "Asbestosis," *Canadian Medical Association Journal* 73 (August 1955): 210.

43 D.C. Braun to H.M. Jackson, August 23, 1957, "Asbestos Chronology," ACRF, 94.

44 Daniel C. Braun and David Truan, "Draft of QAMA: An Epidemiological Study of Lung Cancer in Asbestos Miners," QAMA, 1957, 52.

45 Ibid., 77.

46 Daniel C. Braun and David Truan, "An Epidemiological Study of Lung Cancer in Asbestos Miners," *AMA Archives of Industrial Health* 17 (June 1958): 31–33.

47 Ibid., 74.

48 Kenneth Smith to Yvan Sabourin, C-JM and QAMA Attorney, December 30, 1957, QAMA, 2.

49 Herbert E. Stokinger, AMA, to D.C. Braun, 1958, ACRF.

50 Schepers, "Chronology," 602–3.

51 JM print advertisements, 1958.

52 J.R.M. Hutcheson, C-JM, to G.S. Smith, JMHQ, October 16, 1959, "Asbestos Chronology," ACRF, 104.

53 Corn, *Response to Occupational Health Hazards*, 104.
54 Keal, "Asbestosis and Abdominal Neoplasms," 1211.
55 This information is based on a thorough study of the *Canadian Medical Association Journal* and *Laval medical* throughout their publication history. See, J.D.M., "Asbestosis," 219; Davey and Martin, "Malignant Fibrous Mesothelioma," 792; Haust and Kipkie, "Pleural Mesothelioma," 918.
56 C.B. Burnett, JM President, to JM Managers, July 19, 1960, "Asbestos Chronology," ACRF, 109.
57 Kenneth Smith Presentation to JM Headquarters and General Managers, October 17, 1961, "Asbestos Chronology," ACRF, 107.
58 Selikoff, Churg, and Hammond, "Asbestos Exposure and Neoplasia," 146.
59 Ibid., 145.
60 Kenneth Smith to C.W. Hite, JM, October 13, 1964, "Asbestos Chronology," ACRF, 122.
61 Asbestos Textile Institute Meeting Minutes, June 4, 1965, ACRF, 3.
62 For more information on asbestos and product liability law in the United States, see Barry I. Castleman, *Asbestos: Medical and Legal Aspects*, 5th ed. (New York: Aspen Publishers, 2005), 852.
63 "The Association of Asbestos and Malignancy," 1034.
64 W. Hodgson, C-JM, to A. Pocius, JM, February 1, 1965, "Asbestos Chronology," ACRF, 124.
65 E.C. Lindstrom, JM, to C.H. Jensen, JM, February 12, 1965, "Asbestos Chronology," ACRF, 124.
66 McCulloch and Tweedale, *Defending the Indefensible*, 97.
67 John Beattie, QAMA Meeting Minutes, December 15, 1965, QAMA, 2.
68 Anjivel and Thurlbeck, "The Incidence of Asbestos Bodies," 1179.
69 Tremblay, "Trois cas de néoplasie," 370.
70 QAMA Meeting Minutes, August 10, 1967, QAMA, 44.
71 Ibid., 38; QAMA Meeting Minutes, March 1968, QAMA, 3.
72 QAMA Meeting Minutes, March 1968, QAMA, 3.
73 Employees refused to wear respirators until JM made it mandatory in 1975. See, JM Memo, August 11, 1975, "Asbestos Chronology," ACRF, 167.
74 W.D. Brennan, Tilo Co., to C-JM, November 19, 1968, "Asbestos Chronology," ACRF, 127; Asbestos Fibre Importers Committee, London, to JM and QAMA, October 23, 1968, "Asbestos Chronology," ACRF, 135.
75 Eternit to D. Poutiatine, JM VP Internal, December 22, 1969, "Asbestos Chronology," ACRF, 138.
76 D. Poutiatine to G.E. Parker, "Memo: Labelling of Asbestos and Asbestos-Containing Products for Export Sales," January 25, 1972, "Asbestos Chronology," ACRF, 158.
77 J.R.M. Hutcheson, C-JM, to Swallow, JM, April 27, 1970, "Asbestos Chronology," ACRF, 147.
78 H.M. Jackson to Drs. G.W. Wright and T.H. Davidson, March 17, 1971, "Asbestos Chronology," ACRF, 153.
79 Canadian Johns-Manville to Dr. T.H. Davidson, February-March 1970, "Asbestos Chronology," ACRF, 146.
80 C-JM to T.H. Davidson, February 1970, "Asbestos Chronology," ACRF 138; Reitze to Paul Kotin, JM Health, Safety and Environment VP, July 11, 1978, "Asbestos Chronology," 175.
81 "Poussière à Vendre, Rue Bourbeau," *Le Citoyen*. July 13, 1971, 1. English translation by author.

82 Castleman, 270.
83 JM Asbestos Fiber Division, "Dust Survey of Canadian Asbestos Dust Stations Over TLV," April 24, 1972, "Asbestos Chronology," ACRF, 159.
84 Ibid.
85 John Corbett McDonald, McGill University, "Report," 1972, QAMA, 4–9.
86 Dr. Irving J. Selikoff to Paul C. Formby, December 18, 1972, Irving J. Selikoff Papers.
87 "JM Annual Report, 1973," 12.
88 McDonald and McDonald, "Epidemiologic Surveillance," 359.
89 QAMA Meeting Minutes, January 24, 1974, QAMA, 5.
90 Ibid., 6.
91 The francophone medical community in Quebec during the 1970s was devoted to its professional development rather than to any particular disease or issue. Most of its journal articles at this time were focused on political and developmental issues. See, for example, *La vie médicale au Canada français*, January 1972, 1.
92 J.C. McDonald and Gloria Menard, "Midday Magazine," CBC Radio, March 7, 1974, Irving J. Selikoff Papers (transcript).
93 Turiaf and Battesti, "Le rôle de l'agression asbestosique," 653.
94 Walter Cooper to Paul Kotin, July 29, 1975, "Asbestos Chronology," ACRF, 166.
95 Ibid., 166.
96 David Robertson, *Hard as the Rock Itself* (Boulder: University of Colorado Press, 2011), 10.
97 J.H. Smith, G. Schreiber, L. Eainton, and P. Bergeron, "Report of the Asbestosis Working Group: Subcommittee on Environmental Health" (Ottawa: Health and Welfare Canada, 1975), 10.
98 JM Annual Report, 1975, ACRF, 2.
99 JM Memo, August 11, 1975, "Asbestos Chronology," ACRF, 167.
100 Although health insurance was one of the demands made by Jeffrey Mine workers, a reduction in the levels of dust they were exposed to was not. "Strike 75-123, February 1975," Department of Labour, Strikes and Lockouts, LAC, RG 27, vol. 468, 1.
101 JM Annual Report, 1976, ACRF, 19.
102 R. Beaudry, G. Lagace, and L. Jukau, *Rapport Final: Comite d'Etude sur la Salubrite dans l'Industrie de l'Amiante*, Le Comite, Quebec, 1976.
103 Paul Kotin, September 20, 1977, "Asbestos Chronology," ACRF, 173.
104 JM Executive Bulletin No. E772–2, November 15, 1977, "Asbestos Chronology," ACRF, 174.
105 CBC Radio, 1978, Irving J. Selikoff Papers.
106 *JM Today*, 1980, 2, 3, 2.
107 Ibid., 7.
108 Ibid., 7.
109 Ibid., 7.
110 Hugh Jackson, JM, March 13, 1981, "Asbestos Chronology," ACRF 188–89.
111 "Asbestos, Health and Johns-Manville," 1981, ACRF, 3.
112 Castleman, *Asbestos*, 3.
113 Anna Pirskowski v. Johns-Manville, U.S. District Court, New Jersey, May 28, 1929, "Asbestos Chronology," ACRF, 1.
114 Liddell, "Asbestos and Public Health," 237.
115 James Kelly, "Manville's Bold Maneuver," *Time*, September 6, 1982.

CHAPTER 8: ALTERED AUTHORITY, 1949-83

1 Environment Canada, "Consultation Document: Addition of Chrysotile Asbestos to the PIC Procedure of the Rotterdam Convention" (Government of Canada, 2004): 7.
2 McCulloch and Tweedale, *Defending the Indefensible*, 226.
3 Martin Mittelstaedt, "Asbestos Shame," *The Globe and Mail*, October 27, 2007, 1.
4 "Asbestos Makeover Reignites Old Battle," *Toronto Star*, November 22, 2003, A01.
5 *L'Asbestos*, July 8, 1949 1.
6 Lewis H. Brown, C-JM President, to JM Asbestos Employees, July 19, 1949, Société d'histoire d'Asbestos, 1.
7 Lewis H. Brown, C-JM President, to Mgr. Maurice Roy, Archbishop of Quebec, July 19, 1949, pp. 1–2, Société d'histoire d'Asbestos.
8 Brown to Employees at the Jeffrey Mine, July 19, 1949, Société d'histoire d'Asbestos, 1.
9 $880 once financial aid given was taken into account. Maurice Sauvé, "Six Years Later," in Trudeau, *The Asbestos Strike*, 289.
10 *L'Asbestos*, July 22, 1949, 1.
11 *L'Asbestos*, August 12, 1949, 1.
12 "J'ai 20 ans, j'avais 1 ans et demi de service et j'ai besoin de travailler. Je n'ai pas de mauvais raports avec la compagnie. Je voudrais savoir s'ils vont tous nous reprende où s'ils nous font attendre pour rien. Mon père a une grosse famille et une maison à payer et je suis seul pour l'aider. Je payais pour mon frère de 16 ans qui fait des études pour devenir religieux." English translation by author. Bertrand McNeil to Antonio Barrette, Quebec Minister of Labour, August 19, 1949, BANQ, P659 7C 018 05–02–008B-01; 1982–11–008\1.
13 Gérard Tremblay, sous-ministre du Travail, to Bertrand McNeil, August 22, 1949, BANQ, P659 7C 018 05–02–008B-01; 1982–11–008\1.
14 "Vous allez peut-être me trouver exigeant mais vous savez j'ai un coeur de maman et lorsque je vois mes enfants sans ouvrage cela me peine beaucoup de voir les briseurs de grève pour la plus part faire souffrir des femmes et enfants des grévistes… c'est un grand malheur pour Asbestos que cette triste grève." English translation by author. Mde Eugène Tourigny to Antonio Barrette, Quebec Minister of Labour, September 8, 1949, BANQ, P659 7C 018 05–02–008B-01; 1982–11–008\1.
15 *Procès-verbal*, La ville d'Asbestos, October 5, 1949, 79.
16 *L'Asbestos*, November 29, 1949 1; December 20, 1949, 24.
17 Lampron, Cantin, and Grimard, *Asbestos*, 238.
18 *Procès-verbal*, La ville d'Asbestos, February 15, 1950, 108.
19 *L'Asbestos*, February 21, 1950, 1.
20 *L'Asbestos*, February 28, 1950, 1; Jacques Casgrath, Conseiller to Louis Coderre, Sous-Ministre, M de l'Industrie et du Commerce, August 24, 1951, BANQ, BANQ, P659 7C 018 05–02–008B-01; 1982–11–008\1, and *America*, April 8, 1950, 3.
21 *Le Citoyen*, April 11, 1950, 1.
22 *Le Citoyen*, May 16, 1950, 2.
23 *Le Citoyen*, October 31, 1950, 1.
24 *Procès-verbal*, La ville d'Asbestos, November 29, 1950, 172.
25 "C'est tranquille, dit-on, à Asbestos." English translation by author. *Le Citoyen*, February 27, 1951, 1.
26 *Le Citoyen*, May 15, 1951, 1.
27 *Le Citoyen*, August 31, 1951, 8.

28 Suavé, "Six Years Later," 284.

29 *Le Citoyen*, July 28, 1952, 1.

30 "Parlez-nous de la grève!" and "La grève, c'est une affaire réglée, mon garcon." English translation by author. *Le Citoyen*, July 11, 1952, 1.

31 "Duplessis a plus que prouvé son aversion pour la classe ouvrière…Si vous, travailleurs, le reportez au pouvoir, vous serez en lutte ouverte avec le gouvernement … Mais il y a un jour par 4 ou 5 ans où les ouvriers sont les maîtres, où ils sont les plus forts." English translation by author. *Le Citoyen,* July 11, 1952, 1.

32 *Le Citoyen*, August 8, 1952, 1.

33 *Le Citoyen*, November 7, 1952, 1.

34 "Mon fils, il est vrais que je porte des habits de travail, et que je me souille les mains. Mais, n'aies pas honte de dire bien haut à tes compagnons que la fibre d'amiante, que j'aide à usiner et à manufacturer, joue un rôle dans l'industrie nationale et mondiale." English translation by author. *Entre Nous* (Canadian Johns-Manville Company, May 1955), 3.

35 Pierre Trudeau, "Epilogue," *The Asbestos Strike*, 344–45.

36 Sauvé, "Six Years Later," 280.

37 See for example, André Laurendeau, "Sur cent pages de Pierre Elliott Trudeau," *Le Devoir*, October 6–11, 1956; Cousineau, "Le Sens d'une Grève."

38 "n'est pas sur les résultats de la grève que le débat entre chercheurs va se faire … Nous souhaitons plutôt apporter une attention particulière au débat local, voir en quoi ce conflit va modeler la conscience collective des gens d'Asbestos." English translation by author. Lampron et al., 222.

39 *Procès-verbal*, La ville d'Asbestos, August 6, 1958, 198; August 5, 1959.

40 For more on the FLQ, please see Louis Fournier, *FLQ: Histoire d'un mouvement clandestine*, ed. Edward Baxter (Montreal: Lanctôt Éditeur, 1998); Gérard Pelletier, The October Crisis (Toronto: McClelland and Stewart, 1971).

41 Vallières, *White Niggers of America*, 41.

42 "pendant la grève sànglante de l'amiante." English translation by author. *Le Devoir*, June 18, 1960, 1.

43 *Le Citoyen*, September 27, 1962, 1.

44 Quebec Asbestos Mining Association, QAMA Meeting Minutes, December 14–15, 1965, QAMA, 2.

45 Quebec Asbestos Mining Association, QAMA Meeting Minutes, March 1968, QAMA, 8.

46 *Procès-verbal*, La ville d'Asbestos, April 8, 1969.

47 *Le Citoyen*, December 28, 1974, 204.

48 Quebec Ministry of Natural Resources, "1972 Report," 1, QAMA.

49 J.C. McDonald, McGill University, to CSN, October 25, 1974, QAMA.

50 *Le Citoyen*, December 28, 1974, 114.

51 "on peut dire qu'un tel conflit devient quelque chose de spectaculaire." English translation by author, Ibid., 114.

52 Pierre Trudeau, *Le Citoyen,* December 28, 1974, 3.

53 *Le Citoyen*, December 28, 1974, 210.

54 Department of Labour/Strikes and Lockouts, Strike75–123, LAC, RG 27, vol. 3634, February 1975.

55 *Procès-verbal*, La ville d'Asbestos, October 6, 1976.

56 J.A. McKinney, C-JM President, to René Lévesque, Premier of Quebec, February 14, 1977, BANQ, E78 S999 7A 009 03–06–004B-01; 1993–06–004\12.

57 Michel Carpentier, le chef de Cabinet Adjoint, to Jeannot Picard, CSD, April 28, 1977, BANQ, E78 S999 7A 009 03–06–004B-01; 1993–06–004\12.
58 Morton, *Working People*, 292.
59 J.A. McKinney, C-JM President, to René Lévesque, Premier of Quebec, October 24, 1974, BANQ, E78 S999 7D 024 02–01–001A-01; 1985–02–006\2.
60 *Canadian Mining Journal*, February 1978, 132.
61 J.R.M. Hutcheson, C-JM Administrative Council, to Yves Bérubé, Quebec Minister of the Environment, June 11, 1979, BANQ, E78 S999 7D 024 02–01–001A-01; 1985–02–006\2.
62 C-JM to D. Perlstein, Société nationale de l'amiante President, June 17, 1980, BANQ, E78 S999 7D 024 02–01–001A-01; 1985–02–006\2.
63 Jean-Guy Léger to Yves Bérubé, Quebec Minister of the Environment, August 25, 1980, BANQ, E78 S999 7D 024 02–01–001A-01; 1985–02–006\2.
64 Vallières, *Des Mines et des Hommes*, 367.
65 Kazan-Allen, "Canadian Asbestos," 38.
66 *Procès-verbal*, La ville d'Asbestos, February 16, 1982, 108.
67 *Procès-verbal*, La ville d'Asbestos, March 2, 1982, 114.
68 *Procès-verbal*, La ville d'Asbestos, June 1, 1982, 154; *Canadian Mining Journal*, July 1982, 19.
69 *Procès-verbal*, La ville d'Asbestos, January 4, 1983, 247.
70 *Procès-verbal*, La ville d'Asbestos,1 February 1, 1983, 13.
71 *Procès-verbal*, La ville d'Asbestos, April 19, 1983, 50; May 17, 1983, 63.

Conclusion

1 "Quebec cancer walk nixed over asbestos spat," CBC News, 6 July 2010. http://www.cbc.ca/news/canada/montreal/quebec-cancer-walk-nixed-over-asbestos-spat-1.905987. The Canadian Cancer Society provides financial support, group therapy, and palliative care to many community members dying of asbestos-related cancers.
2 Ibid.
3 See, for example, "Asbestos Makeover Reignites Old Battle," *Toronto Star*, November 22, 2003, A1; Martin Mittelstaedt, "Asbestos Shame," *Globe and Mail*, October 27, 2007, A1; Kathleen Ruff, "Deathbed Reprieve for Killer Industry?" *Toronto Star*, June 6, 2010, 1.
4 For more information on these communities, see Angus and Griffin, *We Lived a Life and Then Some*; Wallace, *St. Clair*; Amundson, *Yellowcake Towns*.
5 "Singing coal miners dig for new talent," CBC News, May 3, 2010, http://www.cbc.ca/news/canada/nova-scotia/singing-coal-miners-dig-for-new-talent-1.911021.
6 See for example, Harold Innis, *The Fur Trade in Canada: An Introduction to Canadian Economic History*, Rev. ed. (Toronto: University of Toronto Press, 1999); Innis, *Staples, Markets, and Cultural Change: Selected Essays*, Rev. ed., ed. Daniel Drache (Montreal and Kingston: McGill–Queen's University Press, 1995).

Bibliography

Note: I engage with a diverse source base in order to provide a nuanced analysis of a single place caught up in a global industry, including local newspaper reports, town council minutes, and JM's corporate archives, located at the worker's compensation litigation-based Asbestos Claims Research Facility (ACRF) in Aurora, Colorado. JM legal counsel assembled some of these sources, such as the "Asbestos Chronology," in order to train new company attorneys in the practices of occupational health lawsuits. These are valuable sources that provide a fascinating examination of how JM dealt with the issues of asbestos-related disease in the town of Asbestos and around the world. Esteemed scholars of the asbestos trade, David Egilman and Geoffrey Tweedale, provided me with many of these documents, and several others have used these sources in previous studies of the global asbestos industry. By engaging with these sources, this book provides an analysis of land, risk, and place over the nineteenth and twentieth centuries, and addresses issues of power and knowledge in relation to how humans interact with the natural environment, and one another.

ARCHIVAL SOURCES

Bibliothèque et Archives nationals du Québec, Quebec City, Quebec, Canada-Fonds Antonio Barrette, P182 3A 017 03-01-003B-01; 2000-10-013\3.
—. Fonds Ministère de la Culture, des Communications et de la Condition feminine, "Industries de Guerre," E8 7A 021 03-05-001B-01; 1960-01-040\183 e24.
—. Fonds Ministère des Ressources naturelles et de la Faune, E78 S999, 7A 009 03-06-004B-01; 1993-06-004\12.
—. Fonds Ministère des Ressources naturelles et de la Faune, E78 S999, 7D 024 02-01-001A-01; 1985-02-006\2.
—. Fonds Ministère des Ressources naturelles et de la Faune, E78 S999, 2A 026 02-05-004A-01; 1993-05-005\4.
—. Fonds René Chaloult, P659 7C 018 05-02-008B-01; 1982-11-008\1.
—. Fonds Société nationale de l'amiante, E69 3A 017 03-07-005A-01; 1989-03-005 1.

Eastern Townships Research Centre, Sherbrooke, Quebec, Canada–W.G. Clarke Fonds
Johns-Manville Claims Resolution Management Corporation, Asbestos Claims Research Facility, Denver, Colorado, United States of America–Asbestos, Quebec Fonds.
La ville d'Asbestos, Asbestos, Quebec, Canada–Procès–verbal.
Library and Archives Canada, Ottawa, Ontario, Canada-Department of Labour, Strikes and Lockouts, RG 27, Vol. 330, Reel T-2713.
–. Department of Labour, Strikes and Lockouts, RG 27, Vol. 381, Reel T-2990.
–. Department of Labour, Strikes and Lockouts, RG 27, Vol. 440, Reel T-4072.
–. Department of Labour, Strikes and Lockouts, RG 27, Vol. 443, Reel T-4076.
–. Department of Labour, Strikes and Lockouts, RG 27, Vol. 444, Reel T-4076.
–. Department of Labour, Strikes and Lockouts, RG 27, Vol. 445, Reel T-4077.
–. Department of Labour, Strikes and Lockouts, RG 27, Vol. 461, Reel T-4092.
–. Department of Labour, Strikes and Lockouts, RG 27, Vol. 468.
–. Department of Labour, Strikes and Lockouts, RG 27, Vol. 3590.
–. Department of Labour, Strikes and Lockouts, RG 27, Vol. 3634.
–. Louis St-Laurent Fonds, MG 26-L, Vol. 56, file I-25-3-A.
Mount Sinai Hospital Archives, New York City – Irving J. Selikoff Papers.
Société d'histoire d'Asbestos, Asbestos, Quebec, Canada.
Turner & Newall Archives, Manchester, England.
Quebec Asbestos Mining Association (QAMA) Fonds.

GOVERNMENT RECORDS

Canada

Canadian Legislative Assembly. "An Act to Incorporate the Canada Central Railway Industry." Session 3, 6th Parliament, Bill 161. Ottawa: Canadian Legislative Assembly, April 12, 1860.
Dominion of Canada Legislature. "First Report of the Special Committee Appointed to Inquire into the Causes Which Retard the Settlement of the Eastern Townships of Lower Canada." Toronto: Lovell and Gibson, 1851.
Environment Canada. "Consultation Document: Addition of Chrysotile Asbestos to the PIC Procedure of the Rotterdam Convention." Government of Canada, 2004.
"Geological Survey of Canada: Report for the Year 1885." Montreal: Dawson Brothers, 1885.
"Geological Survey of Canada: Report for the Year 1886." Montreal: Dawson Brothers, 1886.
"Geological Survey of Canada: Report for the Year 1887." Montreal: Dawson Brothers, 1887.
"Geological Survey of Canada, Report for the Year 1888-1889." Montreal: Dawson Brothers, 1888-1889.
"Geological Survey of Canada: Report for the Year 1902-1903." Montreal: Dawson Brothers, 1903.
"Geological Survey of Canada: Report for the Year 1904." Ottawa: King's Printer, 1904.
"Geological Survey of Canada: Report for the Year 1909." Ottawa: King's Printer, 1909.
"Geological Survey of Canada: Report for the Year 1916." Ottawa: King's Printer, 1916.
"Geological Survey of Canada: Report for the Year 1919." Ottawa: King's Printer, 1919.
Klein, L.A. "Geological Survey of Canada: Report for the Year 1890–1891." Montreal: Dawson Brothers, 1891.
Logan, W.E. "Geological Survey of Canada: Report of Progress for the Year 1847–48." Canadian Geological Survey. Montreal: Lovell and Gibson, 1849.

Murray, Alexander. "Report of Alexander Murray, Esq., Assistant Provincial Geologist, Addressed to W.E. Logan, Esq., Provincial Geologist." Canadian Geological Survey. Montreal: Lovell and Gibson, 1849.

Smith, J.H., G. Schreiber, L. Eainton, and P. Bergeron. "Report of the Asbestosis Working Group: Subcommittee on Environmental Health." Ottawa: Health and Welfare Canada, 1975.

United States of America

Boas, Feodor. "Artificial Stone." United States Patent Office, ed. Washington: 1901.

–. "Composition of Matter for Wall-Plaster." United States Patent Office, ed. Washington: 1896.

Department of the Interior, Bureau of Mines. "1950 Materials Survey: Asbestos." National Security Resources Board Materials Office, ed., 1952.

Quebec

Annuaire Statistique de Québec. E.E. Cinq-Mars, Imprimeur de Le Majesté le Roi, 1914.

Beaudry, R., G. Lagace, L. Jukau. Rapport Final: Comite d'Étude sur la Salubrité dans l'Industrie de l'Amiante. Le Comité, Quebec, 1976.

Déclarations sur la Brutalité de la Police Provinciale à Asbestos, Re: Grève de l'amiante. Sherbrooke: District judicaire d'Arthabaska, 1949.

Institut National de Santé Publique du Québec. "The Epidemiology of Asbestos-Related Diseases in Quebec." Quebec: Insitut National de Santé Publique du Québec, 2004.

Laliberté, Roger. "The Jeffrey Mine of Canadian Johns-Manville Co., Limited, Asbestos, Quebec, Canada." Québec: Ministère des Ressources naturelles et de la Faune, (1972): 1–25.

PERIODICALS

America (1950).

L'Asbestos (1943–55).

The Canadian Mining and Mechanical Review (1890–97).

The Canadian Mining Journal (1949–84).

The Canadian Mining Review (1893–1907).

Le Citoyen (1955–84).

Le Devoir (1949, 1956, 1960, 1997).

Entre Nous (1951–55).

Gazette (Montreal) (1923, 1937).

Globe and Mail (1949, 1997, 2007).

Johns-Manville News Pictorial (1938–59).

Johns-Manville Photo (1938–49).

JM Today (1980).

New York Times (1974).

Ottawa Morning Citizen (1937).

La Patrie (1949).

La Presse (1949).

Quebec Chronicle Telegram (1937).

Richmond Guardian (1892).
Sherbrooke Daily Record (1901, 1909).
Sherbrooke La Tribune (1912).
Time Magazine (1946).
Toronto Clarion (1937).
Toronto Star (1949, 2003, 2010).
Toronto Telegram (1937).
Le Travail (1949).
La Tribune (1918, 1919, 1949).
United States Minerals Yearbook (1937–46)
Winnipeg Manitoba Commonwealth (1937).

OTHER SOURCES – SECONDARY

A.G.N. "Pollution of the Air." *Canadian Medical Association Journal* 22, 4 (1930): 553–54.
Agnew, Harvey. "The Reduction of Noise in Hospitals." *Canadian Medical Association Journal* 23 3 (1930): 417.
Amundson, Michael A. *Yellowcake Towns: Uranium Mining Communities in the American West.* Boulder: University Press of Colorado, 2002.
Andrews, Thomas G. *Killing for Coal: America's Deadliest Labor War.* Cambridge, MA: Harvard University Press, 2008.
Angus, Charlie, and Brit Griffin. *We Lived a Life and Then Some: The Life, Death, and Life of a Mining Town.* Toronto: Between the Lines, 1996.
Anjivel, Lily, and W.M. Thurlbeck. "The Incidence of Asbestos Bodies in the Lungs of Random Necropsies in Montreal." *Canadian Medical Association Journal* 95 (December 3, 1966): 1179–82.
Armstrong, Robert. "Le développement des droits miniers au Québec à la fin du XIXe siècle" [The Development of Mining Rights in Quebec at the end of the 19th Century] *L'Actualite Economique* 59, 3 (September 1983): 576–95. http://dx.doi.org/10.7202/601066ar.
"Asbestos Makeover Reignites Old Battle," *Toronto Star*, November 22, 2003, A01.
"Asbestos Mine Workers to Build Reserve Fund," *CBC News*, June 14, 2010. http://www.cbc.ca/news/canada/montreal/asbestos-mine-workers-to-build-reserve-fund-1.911473.
Becker and Haag Berlin. *Asbestos: Its Sources, Extraction, Preparation, Manufacture, and Uses in Industry and Engineering.* Berlin: Becker and Haag, 1928.
"Asbestos: Where We Live and Work," *Johns-Manville News Pictorial* (October 1950): 8–13.
"Asbestos for Heart Trouble," *Asbestos Magazine* (March 1950): 3.
"Asbestos Production Limited as Strike Continues." *Johns-Manville News Pictorial* (June 1949): 2.
Ashworth, G.J., and Brian Graham, eds. *Senses of Place: Senses of Time, Heritage, Culture and Identity*, Aldershot: Ashgate, 2005.
"The Association of Asbestos and Malignancy." *Canadian Medical Association Journal* 92 (May 8, 1965): 1034–33.
Barrette, Antonio. *Memoirs.* Translated by Marc Sormont. Montreal: Librarie Beauchemin, 1966.
Basso, Keith H. *Wisdom Sits in Places: Landscape and Language among the Western Apache.* Albuquerque: University of New Mexico Press, 1996.

Beaudry, R., G. Lagace, and L. Jukau. *Rapport Final: Comite d'Étude sur la Salubrité dans l'Industrie de l'Amiante*. Le Comite, Québec, 1976.

Beck, Ulrich. *Risk Society: Towards a New Modernity*. Translated by Mark Ritter. London: Sage, 1992.

Behiels, Michael D. *Prelude to Quebec's Quiet Revolution: Liberalism versus Neo-Nationalism, 1945–1960*. Montreal and Kingston: McGill–Queen's University Press, 1985.

–, ed. *Quebec Since 1800: Selected Readings – New Canadian Readings*. Toronto: Irwin Publishing, 2002.

Belshaw, John Douglas. *Colonization and Community: The Vancouver Island Coalfield and the Making of the British Columbian Working Class*. Montreal, Kingston: McGill-Queen's University Press, 2002.

Berman, Daniel M. *Death on the Job: Occupational Health and Safety Struggles in the United States*. New York: Monthly Review Press, 1980.

Black, Conrad. *Duplessis*. Toronto: McClelland and Stewart, 1977.

Booth, J. Derek. *Les Cantons de la Saint-François/Townships of the St. Francis*. Montreal: McCord Museum, McGill University, 1984.

Bourassa, Henri. *Great Britain and Canada: Topics of the Day*. Montreal: C.O. Beauchemin and Fils, 1902.

Bowles, Oliver, and F.M. Barsigian. "Asbestos." In *Minerals Yearbook 1943*. Edited by E.W. Pehrson and C.E. Needham. Washington: US GPO, 1943, 1431.

Bowles, Oliver, and M.A. Cornthwaite. "Asbestos." In *Minerals Yearbook 1937*. Edited by Herbert H. Hughes. Washington: US GPO, 1937, 1368.

Bowles, Oliver, and Dorothy I. Marsh. "Asbestos." In *Minerals Yearbook 1944*. Edited by E.W. Pehrson and C.E. Needham. Washington: United States Printing Office, 1944, 1478.

Bowles, Oliver, and B.H. Stoddard. "Asbestos." In *Minerals Yearbook 1934*. Edited by O.E. Kiessling. Washington: US GPO, 1934, 1014.

Bowles, Oliver, and K.G. Warner. "Asbestos." In *Minerals Yearbook 1939*. Edited by Herbert Hughes. Washington: US GPO, 1939, 1309-10.

Boyle, Peter, Nigel Gray, Jack Henningfield, John Seffrin, and Witold A. Zatonski, eds. *Tobacco: Science, Policy, and Public Health*, 2nd ed. Oxford: Oxford University Press, 2010.

Braun, Daniel C., and David Truan. "An Epidemiological Study of Lung Cancer in Asbestos Miners." *A.M.A. Archives of Industrial Health* 17 (June 1958): 634–53.

British American Land Company. *Lands for Sale in the Eastern Townships of Lower Canada*. London, s.n., 1837.

–. *Lands for Sale in the Eastern Townships of Lower Canada*. London, s.n., 1842.

Brodeur, Paul. *Expendable Americans*. New York: Viking Press, 1974.

–. *Outrageous Misconduct*. New York: Pantheon Books, 1985.

Brown, Lewis H. *La Grève d'Asbestos: Rapport sur le fond de la Question et sur la Position de Canadian Johns-Manville Company, Ltd*. Canadian Johns-Manville, 1949.

Buckley, Karen. *Danger, Death, and Disaster in the Crowsnest Pass Mines, 1902–1928*. Calgary: University of Calgary Press, 2004.

Cameron, Duncan, ed. *Explorations in Canadian Economic History: Essays in Honour of Irene M. Spry*. Ottawa: University of Ottawa Press, 1985.

Carson, Rachel. *Silent Spring*. New York: Houghton Mifflin, 1992 (original work published 1962).

Castleman, Barry I. *Asbestos: Medical and Legal Aspects*, 5th ed. New York: Aspen Publishers, 2005.

–. "Letter to the Editor." *British Journal of Industrial Medicine* 48 (1991): 427–30.

Cirkel, Fritz. *Asbestos: Its Occurrence, Exploitation, and Uses*. Ottawa: Mines Branch, Department of the Interior, 1905.

–. *Chrysotile-Asbestos: Its Occurrence, Exploitation, Milling, and Uses*. Vol. 2. Ottawa: Government Printing Bureau, 1910.

Clark, Claudia. *Radium Girls: Women and Industrial Health Reform, 1910–1935*. Chapel Hill: University of North Carolina Press, 1997.

Clavette, Suzanne. *Les Dessous d'Asbestos: Une Lutte Idéologique Contre la Participation des Travailleurs*. Quebec: Les presses de l'université Laval, 2005.

Cleveland, Edward. *A Sketch of the Early Settlement and History of Shipton, Canada East*. Richmond County Advocate, 1858.

Cooke, W.E. "Fibrosis of the Lungs Due to the Inhalation of Asbestos Dust." *British Medical Journal* 2, 3317 (1924): 147–40. http://dx.doi.org/10.1136/bmj.2.3317.147.

–. "Pulmonary Asbestosis." *British Medical Journal* 2, 3491 (1927): 1024–25.

Cooter, Roger, and John Pickstone, eds. *Medicine in the Twentieth Century*. London: Taylor and Francis, 2000.

Copp, Newton H., and Andrew W. Zanella. *Discovery, Innovation, and Risk: Case Studies in Science and Technology*. Cambridge: MIT Press, 1993.

Corn, Jacqueline Karnell. *Response to Occupational Health Hazards: A Historical Perspective*. New York: Van Nostrand Reinhold, 1992.

Cousineau, Jacques. "Le Sens d'une Grève: Une Interprétation Controuvée." *Relations* (December 1956): 343–46.

Cronon, William. *Changes in the Land: Indians, Colonists, and the Ecology of New England*. New York: Hill and Wang, 1983.

–. *Uncommon Ground: Rethinking the Human Place in Nature*. New York: W.W. Norton, 1995.

–. *Uncommon Ground: Toward Reinventing Nature*, ed. William Cronon. New York: W.W. Norton, 1995.

Davey, P.W., and G.M. Martin. "Malignant Fibrous Mesothelioma of Peritoneum." *Canadian Medical Association Journal* 77 (October 15, 1957): 792.

Day, Catherine Matilda. *History of the Eastern Townships, Province of Quebec, Dominion of Canada, Civil and Descriptive in Three Parts*. Montreal: John Lovell, 1869.

Delisle, Esther, and Pierre K. Malouf. *Le Quatuor d'Asbestos: Autour de la Grève d'Amiante*. Montreal: Les Éditions Varia, 2004.

Delorme, Marie-Josée. *La M.R.C. d'Asbestos: Un Coin de l'Estrie*. Asbestos: Commission Scholaire d'Asbestos, 1991.

Denis, Theo. C. "The Mining Industry in the Province of Quebec in 1919." *Canadian Mining Journal* 41 (January 4, 1920): 4.

Derickson, Alan. *Black Lung: Anatomy of a Public Health Disaster*. Ithaca: Cornell University Press, 1998.

–. *Workers' Health: Workers' Democracy – The Western Miners' Struggle, 1891–1925*. Ithaca: Cornell University Press, 1998.

Desmeules, R., L. Rousseau, M. Giroux, and A. Sirois, "Amiantose et Cancers Pulmonaires," *Laval Médical: Bulletin de la société médicale des hôpitaux universitaires Québec* 6, 3 (March 1941): 97–108.

Diamond, Jared. *Collapse: How Societies Choose to Fail or Succeed.* New York: Viking, 2005.

Dineley, D.L. "Devonian." In *The Oxford Companion to the Earth.* Edited by Paul Hancock and Brian J. Skinner. Oxford: Oxford University Press, 2000. http://www.oxford reference.com.

Dolbec, Michel. "Les marathoniens de l'amiante sont ignores." *Le Devoir,* April 5, 1997, A2.

Doll, Richard. "Mortality from Lung Cancer in Asbestos Workers." *British Journal of Industrial Medicine* 12 (1953).

Douglas, Mary. *Risk and Blame: Essays in Cultural Theory.* London: Routledge, 1992. http://dx.doi.org/10.4324/9780203430866.

–. *Risk and Culture: An Essay on the Selection of Technical and Environmental Dangers.* Berkeley: University of California Press, 1982.

Dresser, John A. "Mining in Quebec." *Canadian Mining Journal* 44 (August 17, 1923): 645.

Dubois, Jean. *The White Plague: Tuberculosis, Man and Society.* New Brunswick: Rutgers University Press, 1987.

Durbach, Nadja. "'They Might as Well Brand Us': Working-Class Resistance to Compulsory Vaccination in Victorian England." *Social History of Medicine* 13, 1 (2000): 45–63.

Egbert, D.S., and A.J. Geiger. "Pulmonary Asbestosis and Carcinoma." *American Review of Tuberculosis* 34 (1936), 143–50.

Egilman, David, Corey Fehnel, and Susanna Rankin Bohme. "Exposing the 'Myth' of ABC: 'Anything but Chrysotile' – A Critique of the Canadian Asbestos Mining Industry and McGill University Chrysotile Studies." *American Journal of Industrial Medicine* 44, 5 (2003): 540–57. http://dx.doi.org/10.1002/ajim.10300.

Egilman, David, and Candace M. Hom. "Corruption of the Medical Literature: A Second Visit." *American Journal of Industrial Medicine* 34, 4 (1998): 401–4. http://dx.doi.org/10.1002/(SICI)1097-0274(199810)34:4<401::AID-AJIM16>3.0.CO;2-6.

English, John. *Citizen of the World: The Life of Pierre Elliott Trudeau, 1919–1968.* Toronto: A.A. Knopf, 2006.

Ericson, Richard V., and Aaron Doyle, eds. *Risk and Morality.* Toronto: University of Toronto Press, 2003.

Ewen, Geoffrey. "The International Unions and the Workers' Revolt in Quebec, 1914–1925." PhD diss., York University, 1998.

Fabien, Frère. *Au Fil des Années: Historique de l'École St-Aimé, 1918–1968.* Sherbrooke: Éditions Paulines, 1968.

Farrar, Margaret E. *Building the Body Politic: Power and Urban Space in Washington, D.C.* Urbana: University of Illinois Press, 2008.

Fish, Richard. "Canadian Johns-Manville Beginning $77 Million Investment Program." *Canadian Mining Journal* 98 (November 1977): 8–11.

Foucault, Michel. *The Birth of the Clinic: An Archaeology of Medical Perception.* New York: Vintage, 1994.

–. *The Order of Things: An Archaeology of the Human Sciences.* New York: Vintage, 1973.

Fournier, Louis. *FLQ: Histoire d'un mouvement clandestine* [The Anatomy of an Underground Movement]. Translated by Edward Baxter. Montreal: Lanctôt Éditeur, 1998.

Gagnon, Alain-G., and Michel Sarra-Bournet, eds. *Duplessis: Entre la Grande Noirceur et la Société Libérale, Program d'Études sur le Québec de l'Université McGill.* Montreal: Éditions Québec Amérique, 1997.

Gatrell, Anthony C., and Susan J. Elliott. *Geographies of Health: An Introduction,* 2nd ed. Malden: Wiley-Blackwell, 2009.

Gesler, William M., and Robin A. Kearns. *Culture/Place/Health*. New York: Routledge, 2002.

Gillies, Elizabeth W. "The Asbestos Industry since 1929 with Special Reference to Canada." M.A. thesis, McGill University, 1941.

Gordon, Linda. *The Great Arizona Orphan Abduction*. Cambridge, MA: Harvard University Press, 1999.

Gray, Alexander. "Asbestos Industry Readjusted." *Canadian Mining Journal* 47 (April 9, 1926): 402.

Greenberg, Morris. "A Report on the Health of Asbestos, Quebec Miners 1940." *American Journal of Industrial Medicine* 48, 3 (2005): 230–37. http://dx.doi.org/10.1002/ajim.20206.

Grenier, Guy. *100 Ans de Médecine: Histoire de l'Association des Médicins de Langue Français de Canada*. Montréal: Éditions MultiMondes, 2002.

Hahn, Michael. "A Clash of Cultures? The UNESCO Diversity Convention and International Trade Law." *Journal of International Economic Law* 9, 3 (September 2006): 515–52. http://dx.doi.org/10.1093/jiel/jgl021.

Hall, Stuart, and Paul Du Gay, eds. *Questions of Cultural Identity*. London: Sage, 2003.

Haust, M. Daria, and G.F. Kipkie. "Pleural Mesothelioma." *Canadian Medical Association Journal* 81 (December 1, 1959): 918.

Heaman, E.A., Alison Li, and Shelley McKellar, eds. *Essays in Honour of Michael Bliss: Figuring the Social*. Toronto: University of Toronto Press, 2008.

Heron, Craig. *The Canadian Labour Movement, A Brief History*. 2nd ed. Toronto: James Lorimer, 1996 (Original work published 1989).

Hogen, Patrick Colm. *Colonialism and Cultural Identity*. Albany: SUNY Press, 2000.

Hovis, Logan, and Jeremy Mouat. "Miners, Engineers, and the Transformation of Work in the Western Mining Industry, 1889–1930." *Technology and Culture* 37, 3 (July 1996): 429–56.

Hueper, W.C. "Silicosis, Asbestosis, and Cancer of the Lung." *American Journal of Clinical Pathology* 25 (December 1955): 1340–88.

Ingold, Tim. *The Perception of the Environment: Essays in Livelihood, Dwelling, and Skill*. London: Routledge, 2000. http://dx.doi.org/10.4324/9780203466025.

Innis, Harold. *The Fur Trade in Canada: An Introduction to Canadian Economic History*. Toronto: University of Toronto Press, Revised Edition, 1999.

–. *Staples, Markets, and Cultural Change: Selected Essays*, Revised Edition. Edited by Daniel Drache. Montreal/Kingston: McGill-Queen's University Press, 1995.

Institut National de Santé Publique du Québec. "The Epidemiology of Asbestos-Related Diseases in Quebec." Quebec: Insitut National de Santé Publique du Québec, 2004.

J.D.M. "Asbestosis." *Canadian Medical Association Journal* 73 (August 1955): 210.

Jacobs, Nancy. *Environment, Power, and Injustice: A South African History*. Cambridge: Cambridge University Press, 2003. http://dx.doi.org/10.1017/CBO9780511511981.

Jameson, Elizabeth. *All That Glitters: Class, Conflict, and Community in Cripple Creek*. Urbana: University of Illinois Press, 1998.

Jones, Richard. *Duplessis and the Union Nationale Administration*. Ottawa: Canadian Historical Association, 1983.

Jones, Robert H. *Asbestos and Asbestic: Their Properties, Occurrence, and Use*. London: Crosby Lockwood and Son, 1897.

–. "Asbestos and Asbestic: With some Account of the Recent Discovery of the Latter at Danville, in Lower Canada." *Canadian Mining Review* 16 (1897): 186–87.

Josephson, G.W., and F.M. Barsigian. "Asbestos." *Minerals Yearbook 1949*. Edited by Allen F. Matthews. Washington: United States Printing Office, 1951. 139–48.

Josephson, G.W., and Dorothy I. Marsh. "Asbestos." In *Minerals Yearbook 1946*. Edited by E.W. Pehrson and Allen F. Matthews. Washington: US GPO, 150.

Judkins, Bennett M. *We Offer Ourselves as Evidence: Toward Workers' Control of Occupational Health*. Westport: Greenwood Press, 1986.

Kazan-Allen, Laurie. *Canadian Asbestos: A Global Concern*. International Ban Asbestos Secretariat, 2003.

Keal, E.E. "Asbestosis and Abdominal Neoplasms." *Lancet* 276, 7162 (December 1960): 1211–16. http://dx.doi.org/10.1016/S0140-6736(60)92413-2.

Kealey, Gregory S. *Workers and Canadian History*. Montreal and Kingston: McGill–Queen's University Press, 1995.

Kelly, James. "Manville's Bold Maneuver." *Time*, September 6, 1982.

Kessner, Thomas. *Capital City: New York City and the Men behind America's Rise to Economic Dominance, 1860–1900*. New York: Simon and Schuster, 2003.

Kesteman, Jean-Pierre, Peter Southam, and Diane Saint-Pierre. *Histoire des Cantons de l'Est*. Sainte-Foy: Les Presses de l'Université Laval, 1998.

Klein, Cornelis. "Rocks, Minerals, and a Dusty World." In *Reviews in Mineralogy: Health Effects of Mineral Dusts*. Edited by Brooke T. Mossman and George D. Guthrie Jr. Chelsea: Mineralogical Society of America, 1993, 17.

Kotkin, Stephen. *Magnetic Mountain: Stalinism as a Civilization*. Berkeley: University of California Press, 1995.

Lamonde, Yvan. *Histoire Sociale des Idées au Québec, 1760–1896*. Vol. 1: *1760–1896*. Vol. 2: *1896–1929*. Montréal: Éditions Fides, 2000.

Lamonde, Yvan, and Claude Corbo, eds. *Le Rouge et le Bleu: Une Anthologie de la Pensée Politique au Québec de la Conquête à la Révolution Tranquille*. Montréal: Les Presses de l'Université de Montreal, 1999.

Lampron, Réjean, Marc Cantin, and Élise Grimard. *Asbestos: Filons D'Histoire, 1899–1999*. Asbestos: Centenaire de la ville d'Asbestos, 1999.

Lankton, Larry. *Cradle to Grave: Life, Work, and Death at the Lake Superior Copper Mines*. Oxford: Oxford University Press, 1991.

Lanza, A.J. "Asbestosis," *Journal of the American Medical Association* 106, 5 (1936): 368–69.

Lapointe, Simon. *L'influence de la Gauche Catholique Française sur l'Idéologie de la CTCC-CSN de 1948–1964*. Montréal: La Collection RCHTQ, 1996.

Lash, Scott, Bronislaw Szerszynski, and Brian Wynne, eds. *Risk, Environment, and Modernity*. London: Sage, 1996.

Latour, Bruno. *Science in Action: How to Follow Scientists and Engineers through Society*. Cambridge, MA: Harvard University Press, 1997.

Leavitt, Judith Walzer. *Typhoid Mary: Captive to the Public's Health*. Boston: Beacon Press, 1995.

LeDoux, Burton. *L'Amiantose: Un Village de Trois Mille Âmes Étouffe dans la Poussière*: East Broughton, 1949.

Létourneau, Jocelyn. "La Grève de l'Amiante Entre ses Mémoires et l'Histoire." *Oral History Forum d'histoire orale* 11 (1991): 8–16.

Levitt, Joseph. *Henri Bourassa and the Golden Calf: The Social Programs of the Nationalists of Quebec (1900–1914)*, 2nd ed. Les Editions de l'Université d'Ottawa, 1972.

–. *Henri Bourassa on Imperialism and Bi-Culturalism, 1900–1918.* Edited by Joseph Levitt. Toronto: Copp Clark, 1970.

Liddell, F.D. "Asbestos and Public Health." *Canadian Medical Association Journal* 125, 3 (September 1981): 237-39.

Linteau, Paul-André, René Durocher, Jean-Claude Robert, et al. *Quebec: A History, 1867–1929.* Translated by Robert Chodos. Toronto: James Lorimer, 1983.

–. *Quebec Since 1930.* Translated by Robert Chodos and Ellen Garmais. Toronto: James Lorimer, 1991.

Little, J.I. *Ethno-Cultural Transition and Regional Identity in the Eastern Townships of Quebec.* Ottawa: Keystone Printing and Lithographing, 1989.

–. *Nationalism, Capitalism, and Colonization in Nineteenth-Century Quebec: The Upper St. Francis District.* Montreal and Kingston: McGill–Queen's University Press, 1980.

Lupton, Deborah. *Risk.* London and New York: Routledge, 1999.

MacDermot, H.E. *History of the Canadian Medical Association,* Vol. 1: *1867–1921.* Toronto: Murray Printing, 1935.

–. *History of the Canadian Medical Association.* Vol. 2. Toronto: Murray Printing and Gravure, 1958.

Maines, Rachel P. *Asbestos and Fire: Technological Trade-Offs and the Body at Risk.* New Brunswick: Rutgers University Press, 2005.

Mann, Susan. *The Dream of a Nation: A Social and Intellectual History of Quebec.* 2nd ed. Montreal and Kingston: McGill–Queen's University Press, 2002 (original work published 1982).

Margai, Florence M., *Environmental Health Hazards and Social Justice: Geographical Perspectives on Race and Class Disparities.* London: Earthscan, 2010.

Markowitz, Gerald, and David Rosner. *Deadly Dust: Silicosis and the Politics of Industrial Disease in Twentieth-Century America.* Princeton: Princeton University Press, 1994.

–. *Deceit and Denial: The Deadly Politics of Environmental Pollution.* Berkeley: University of California Press, 2002.

McAnany, Patricia A., and Norman Yoffee. "Why We Question Collapse and Study Human Resilience, Ecological Vulnerability, and the Aftermath of Empire." In *Questioning Collapse: Human Resilience, Ecological Vulnerability, and the Aftermath of Empire.* Edited by Patricia A. McAnany and Norman Yoffee. Cambridge: Cambridge University Press, 2009.

McCulloch, Jock, and Geoffrey Tweedale. *Defending the Indefensible: The Global Asbestos Industry and Its Fight for Survival.* Oxford: Oxford University Press, 2008.

McDonald, Alison D., and J.C. McDonald. "Epidemiologic Surveillance of Mesothelioma in Canada." *Canadian Medical Association Journal* 109 (September 1, 1973): 359–62.

McRoberts, Kenneth. *Quebec: Social Change and Political Crisis.* Toronto: McClelland and Stewart, 1988.

Merewether, E.R.A. *Annual Report of the Chief Inspector of Factories for the Year 1947.* London: H.M. Stationary office, 1949.

Merewether, E.R.A., and C.W. Price. "A Memorandum on Asbestosis." *Tubercle* 15, 2 (1933): 69–81. http://dx.doi.org/10.1016/S0041-3879(33)80023-7.

Miles, Henry H. *Canada East at the International Exhibition.* London: s.n. 1862.

Morton, Desmond. *Working People.* 3rd ed. Toronto: Summerhill Press, 1990 (original work published 1980).

Mossman, Brooke T., and George D. Guthrie, Jr., eds. *Health Effects of Mineral Dusts.* Reviews in Mineralogy. Chelsea: Mineralogical Society of America, 1993.

Murphy, Michelle. *Sick Building Syndrome and the Problem of Uncertainty*. Durham: Duke University Press, 2006. http://dx.doi.org/10.1215/9780822387831.

Nordmann, M. "The Occupational Cancer of Asbestos Workers." *Z Krebsforsch* 47 (1938), 288–302.

O'Hanley, David S. "The Origin of the Chrysotile Asbestos Veins in Southwestern Quebec." *Canadian Journal of Earth Sciences* 24, 1 (January 1987): 1–9. http://dx.doi.org/10.1139/e87-001.

Obalski, Joseph. *Mines and Minerals of the Province of Quebec*. Quebec: Province of Quebec, 1889.

–. *Province de Québec: Industries Minérales: Préparé Spécialement pour l'Exposition de Liège, Belgique*. Quebec: Dussault and Proulx, 1905.

Ostry, Aleck. *Change and Continuity in Canada's Health Care System*. Ottawa: CHA Press, 2006.

Palmer, Bryan D. *Working-Class Experience: Rethinking the History of Canadian Labour, 1800–1991*. 2nd ed. Toronto: McClelland and Stewart, 1992 (original work published 1983).

Parent, Gilles. *Deux Efforts de Colonisation Française dans les Cantons de l'Est, 1848 et 1851*. Sherbrooke: Librairie Dussault et de René Prince, 1980.

Parr, Joy. *Sensing Changes: Technologies, Environments, and the Everyday*. Vancouver: UBC Press, 2010.

Pedley, Frank G. "Asbestosis." *Canadian Medical Association Journal* 22, 2 (1930): 253.

–. "Review of E.R.A. Merewether, 'Occurrence of Pulmonary Fibrosis and Other Pulmonary Affections in Asbestos Workers.'" *Canadian Medical Association Journal* 23, 6 (1930): 872–73.

–. "Review of 'Pulmonary Asbestosis: Its Clinical, Radiological, and Pathological Features, and Associated Risk of Tuberculosis Infection.'" *Canadian Medical Association Journal* 29, 4 (1933): 448.

–. "Review of Studies in Experimental Pneumonokoniosis, VI. Inhalation of Asbestos Dust: Its Effect Upon Primary Tuberculosis Infection." *Canadian Medical Association Journal* 24, 6 (1931): 883.

Pelletier, Gérard. *The October Crisis*. Toronto: McClelland and Stewart, 1971.

Piper, Liza. *The Industrial Transformation of Subarctic Canada*. Vancouver: UBC Press, 2009.

–. "Subterranean Bodies: Mining the Large Lakes of North-West Canada, 1921–1960." *Environmental History* 13, 2 (2007): 155–86. http://dx.doi.org/10.3197/096734007780473500.

"Quebec Tax on Mining." *Canadian Mining and Mechanical Review* 10, 2 (1891): 31–32.

Rajala, Richard A. *Clearcutting the Pacific Rainforest: Production, Science, and Regulation*. Vancouver: UBC Press, 1998.

Reverby, Susan M. *Examining Tuskegee: The Infamous Syphilis Study and its Legacy*. University of North Carolina Press, 2009.

–, ed. *Rethinking the Tuskegee Syphilis Study*. Chapel Hill: University of North Carolina Press, 2000.

Robertson, David. *Hard as the Rock Itself: Place and Identity in the American Mining Town*. Boulder: University of Colorado Press, 2010.

Rosen, George. *The History of Miners' Diseases: A Medical and Social Interpretation*. New York: Schuman's Press, 1943.

Rosenberg, Charles E. *Explaining Epidemics and Other Studies in the History of Medicine*. Cambridge: Cambridge University Press, 1992. http://dx.doi.org/10.1017/CBO9780511666865.

Ross, W. "Encroachment of the Jeffrey Mine on the Town of Asbestos, Quebec." *Geographical Review* 57, 4 (1967): 523–37. http://dx.doi.org/10.2307/212931.

Rothery, David A. "Obduction." In *The Oxford Companion to the Earth*. Edited by Paul Hancock and Brian J. Skinner. Oxford: Oxford University Press, 2000. http://www.oxfordreference.com.

Rothman, Sheila M. *Living in the Shadow of Death: Tuberculosis and the Social Experience of Illness in American History.* Baltimore: Johns Hopkins University Press, 1995.

Rouillard, Jacques. *L'Expérience Syndicale au Québec: Ses Rapports avec l'État, La Nation et l'Opinion Publique.* Montréal: VLB Éditeur, 2008.

–. "La Grève de l'Amiante, Mythe et Symbolique." *L'Action Nationale (Toulouse)* 89, 7 (September 1999): 33–43.

–. "La Grève de l'Amiante de 1949 et le Projet de Réforme de l'Entreprise. Comment le Patronat a Défendu son Droit de Gérance." *Labour/Le travail* (Fall 2000): 307–42.

–. *Le Syndicalisme Québécois: Deux Siècles d'Histoire.* Montréal: Boréal, 2004.

–. *Les Syndicats Nationaux au Québec de 1900 à 1930.* Québec: Les Cahiers d'histoire de l'université Laval, 1979.

Rousseau, Louis. "Amiantose Pulmonaire." *Laval Medical* 8 (1943): 239.

–. "Quelque considérations sur l'amiantose." *Laval Medical* 11 (1946): 57.

Ruff, Kathleen. "Deathbed Reprieve for Killer Industry?" *Toronto Star*, June 6, 2010.

Ryan, Paul D. "Caledonides." In *The Oxford Companion to the Earth*. Edited by Paul Hancock and Brian J. Skinner. Oxford: Oxford University Press, 2000. http://www.oxfordreference.com.

Schepers, Gerrit W.H. "Chronology of Asbestos Cancer Discoveries: Experimental Studies of the Saranac Laboratory." *American Journal of Industrial Medicine* 27, 4 (1995): 593–606. http://dx.doi.org/10.1002/ajim.4700270413.

"Science Supplement, 3 December 1926.," "Reviews and Retrospects." *Canadian Medical Association Journal* 17, 1 (1927): 93.

Selikoff, I.J., J. Churg, and E.C. Hammond. "Asbestos Exposure and Neoplasia." *Journal of the American Medical Association* 188, 1 (April 1964): 142–46. http://dx.doi.org/10.1001/jama.1964.03060270028006.

Sellers, Christopher C. *Hazards of the Job: From Industrial Disease to Environmental Health Science.* Chapel Hill: University of North Carolina Press, 1997.

"Silicosis." *Canadian Medical Association Journal* (1934): 304.

Sinclair, W.E. *Asbestos: Its Origin, Production, and Utilization.* London: Mining Publications, 1959.

Skinner, H. Catherine W., Malcolm Ross, and Clifford Frondel. *Asbestos and Other Fibrous Minerals.* Oxford: Oxford University Press, 1988, 196, 33.

Smith, Barbara Ellen. *Digging Our Own Graves: Coal Miners and the Struggle over Black Lung Disease.* Philadelphia: Temple University Press, 1987.

Smith, J.H., G. Schreiber, L. Eainton, and P. Bergeron. "Report of the Asbestosis Working Group: Subcommittee on Environmental Health." Ottawa: Health and Welfare Canada, 1975.

Smith, Kenneth. "Pulmonary Disability in Asbestos Workers." *AMA Archives of Industrial Health* 12 (1955): 198–203.

Sparks, J.B. "Pulmonary Asbestosis." *Radiology* 17, 6 (1931): 1249–57. http://dx.doi.org/10.1148/17.6.1249.

Summers, A. Leonard. *Asbestos and the Asbestos Industry: The World's Most Wonderful Mineral and Other Fireproof Materials*. London: Sir Isaac Pitman and Sons, 1920.

Tataryn, Lloyd. *Dying for a Living: The Politics of Industrial Death*. Toronto: Deneau and Greenberg, 1979.

Therrien, A. "Vertical Section A, B, C, Jeffrey Mine Area." Asbestos: Canadian Johns-Manville, 1971.

Tomesco, Frederic. "Asbestos, Quebec, Seeks a Healthier Name Not Linked to Cancer," *Bloomberg.com*, July 14, 2006.

Tremblay, Jean-Paul. "Trois cas de néoplasie associés à de l'amiantose." *Laval Medical* 38 (April 1967): 370–72.

Trudeau, Pierre Elliott, ed. *The Asbestos Strike*. Translated by James Boake. Toronto: James Lewis and Samuel, 1970 (original work published 1956).

"Tuberculose et Amiantose." *Laval Medical* 12 (1947): 1090.

Turiaf, J., and J.P. Battesti. "Le rôle de l'agression asbestosique dans la provocation du mésothéliome pleural." *La Vie Medicale au Canada Francais* 3 (June 1974): 653.

Tweedale, Geoffrey. *Magic Mineral to Killer Dust*. Oxford: Oxford University Press, 2000.

US Environmental Protection Agency. "Environmental Justice." http://www.epa.gov/compliance/environmentaljustice.

Vagt, G.O. "Asbestos." *Canadian Mining Journal*, February 1984, 143.

Vallières, Marc. *Des Mines et des Hommes: Histoire de l'Industrie Minérale Québécoise des Origines au Début des Années 1980*. Québec: Publications du Québec, 1989.

Vallières, Pierre. *White Niggers of America: The Precocious Autobiography of a Quebec Terrorist*. Translated by Joan Pinkham. Toronto: McClelland and Stewart, 1971 (original work published 1966).

Vigod, Bernard L. *Quebec before Duplessis: The Political Career of Louis-Alexandre Taschereau*. Kingston and Montreal: McGill–Queen's University Press, 1986.

Ville d'Asbestos, Québec, Canada. Québec: Ministère des Richesses Naturelles, 1967.

Walkom, L.K. "New Shaft, Unusual New Mill: Feature Expansion at World's Largest Asbestos-Producing Property." *Canadian Mining Journal* 75 (October 1954): 57–58.

Wallace, Anthony F.C. *St. Clair: A Nineteenth-Century Coal Town's Experience with a Disaster-Prone Industry*. 3rd ed. New York: A.A. Knopf, 1987 (original work published 1981).

Wallot, Hubert. "La salubrité dans l'industrie de l'amiante." *La Vie Medicale au Canada Francais* 8 (February 1979): 157

Wallraff, Günter. *Lowest of the Low*. London: Methuen, 1988.

White, Richard. *The Organic Machine: The Remaking of the Columbia River*. New York: Hill and Wang, 1996.

Whiteside, James. *Regulating Danger: The Struggle for Mine Safety in the Rocky Mountain Coal Industry*. Lincoln: University of Nebraska Press, 1990.

Wolff, David A. *Industrializing the Rockies: Growth, Competition, and Turmoil in the Coalfields of Colorado and Wyoming, 1868–1914*. Boulder: University Press of Colorado, 2003.

Zaslow, Morris. *Reading the Rocks: The Story of the Geological Survey of Canada, 1842–1972*. Ottawa: Macmillan, in association with the Department of Energy, Mines and Resources and Information Canada, 1975.

Index

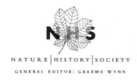

NATURE|HISTORY|SOCIETY

GENERAL EDITOR: GRAEME WYNN

Printed and bound in Canada by Friesens
Set in Garamond by Artegraphica Design Co. Ltd.
Copy editor: Matthew Kudelka
Proofreader: Dianne Tiefensee
Cartographer: Eric Leinberger